Peter Buckland is a grandfather to three boys from his two daughters and remains married (just about). The loss of his son to an incurable disease brought a devastating darkness to his remaining family. Peter felt a compelling need to share this tragedy and try and make a difference within government and the blood transfusion service.

THE WITCHES WITHIN WESTMINSTER

To my late Son, Mark Adam Buckland, who despite knowing he only had a short time to live, spent the last 5 months on this precious earth unselfishly as indeed he had up to his death.

Peter Buckland

THE WITCHES WITHIN WESTMINSTER

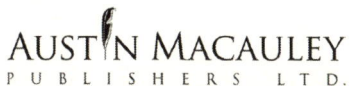

Copyright © Peter Buckland

The right of Peter Buckland to be identified as author of this work has been asserted by him in accordance with section 77 and 78 of the Copyright, Designs and Patents Act 1988.

All rights reserved. No part of this publication may be reproduced, stored in a retrieval system, or transmitted in any form or by any means, electronic, mechanical, photocopying, recording, or otherwise, without the prior permission of the publishers.

Any person who commits any unauthorized act in relation to this publication may be liable to criminal prosecution and civil claims for damages.

A CIP catalogue record for this title is available from the British Library.

ISBN 978 1 84963 756 5

www.austinmacauley.com

First Published (2014)
Austin Macauley Publishers Ltd.
25 Canada Square
Canary Wharf
London
E14 5LB

Printed and bound in Great Britain

Foreword

How do I move forward with grace between the extremes of loving, and having to let go .I've been given a calling, a work of writing I so often couldn't accomplish. When I first announced to my Family that one day I would write a book about my late son's death I must admit I didn't really believe that I ever would. Most nights I still dream of my late son Mark either as a young blonde haired, blue eyed boy, who unlike his dad was blessed with a serenity that few possess, or I can meet with him again in the very winter of his ever so short life pushing his spent body down a one way street in Brighton, his home town.

I am still on that sideline now along with the rest of my family except while we so desperately wanted to get back to the game of leading a normal life, the Witches, the ones within Westminster who took our son's dreams, and our love for him, and buried them in six feet of chalk on the Sussex downs; still remain to haunt our family.

It is only now after many sleepless nights that I have found the mental strength to share this tragedy, and relate this moving story to anyone who ever thought that life was fair, and that the governmental structure within Westminster was a sane and safe, and responsible one.

What you are about to read is strictly factual and I have no fear in being compromised.

For some time I had been looking, searching for a title for this book, and do you know it came to me in a dream, actually most of that dream was more like a nightmare, you will see hopefully just why I chose this title *The witches within Westminster.*

In April 1985 the first known case of B.S.E. was recorded in the UK, however there may have been more unrecorded cases before. Dubbed by the press as [Mad cows disease] some

10 years later this incurable disease had crossed the human species barrier and claimed its first recorded human Victim. In 1995, 18 year old Stephen Churchill died of Human B S E. Referred to now as [New variant vCJD] again it's also very possible there may have been more deaths to vCJD not recorded before or since! In my opinion these figures were manipulated by the Tories and have been ever since, it wasn't after all in their interests to detail the facts or indeed numbers of mortalities due to BSE exposure.

On March 20th 1996 the then Tory Health Minister Stephen Dorrell, announced in Parliament that 10 people under the age of 42 had died from new variant CJD.

In 2010, that human death toll has risen to 177 and rising [although again it may well be more!]

The responsibility for the Murder of these Innocent victims it could be said were those ministers who from 1979 deregulated the Beef industry. Under Margaret Thatcher's newly formed government it was her wish to let the "market decide" This Thatcher philosophy had terrible consequences for safety standards within the UK Abbotairs, now under pressure from the feed suppliers and the banks, farmers had begun to use feed derived from animal carcasses to include cows to feed cattle. After the 1974 Middle East war the price of oil escalated, rather than Grain, MAAF decided that to convert cows into carnivores would be a good idea; an enormous cost saving exercise for the UK government in grain and hay, but at what cost!

A relaxation in the temperature and manufacturing techniques of rendering processes within Abbotairs was a direct result of incoming Prime Minister Margaret Thatcher's policies in 1979 ,and may have led to BSE and eventually vCJD. The temperatures were lowered from 150 deg to an unspecified amount, there was also a cessation in the rendering process in the use of solvent extractors, such as acetone, to recover the last scraps of meat. All researchers agree however that the recycling of cows to feed other cows amplified the BSE agent, in 1988 Wilesmith and colleagues demonstrated the role of meat and bone meal in the onset of the BSE epidemic, they also in 1991 through their studies suggested that BSE – agent transmission through meat and bone meal could result, from halting the use of organic solvents in the manufacturing and rendering process. The food industry is Big Business; Supermarkets like Sainsbury's, Asda and Tesco dominate the marketplace. To increase profits they must compete with one another to pressurise their suppliers, the renderers, slaughterers and certainly the farmers. To defend their business interests they did go to any lengths, and it continued into John Major's Tory govt, [MAAF], [1]The ministry of health, in fact all of the other Govt Departments who deceived the public to hide the crisis, including those Parliamentary Parties who never acted despite the detailed evidence that lay before them. They were blinded by increased profit margins, blinkered to the already known dangers of Cannibalism. Prion diseases are warning us that something is out of balance, that the excessive unnaturalness we force on livestock has finally come to destroy mankind.

IN short the Government and its associated scientific advisors sabotaged science, the cause of BSE and its associated cross over to the human species in vCJD was the introduction of the cannibalistic forced feeding of cattle. For the dairy herds this witches' brew was a protein mix of, amongst other offal, the ground up brains and spinal cord of other cattle, these parts were among the most infectious.

This Witches' brew was named as (SBO) specified bovine offal, then fed back to both dairy and some beef herds in the form of [MBM]- short for meat bone meal, and it needed to be mixed with Molasses as a sweetener, in order to make it palatable for the milking herds. And why you may ask? A mad scramble for Profit, in the milking parlours a Greater yield, but at what human cost? The political philosophy of the then Prime Minister, Margaret Thatcher, was predicated on the assumption that, other things being equal, the state should intervene as rarely as possible in market transactions and that

---

[1] The term MAAF meaning the ministry of agriculture and fisheries.

the proportion of the Gross National Product spent by the state should be diminished; in essence acting like Dickens' Scrooge.

Thatcherite macro-economic policy favoured a [laissez faire] approach to consumer and environmental protection, but in the early 1980's at any rate the UK government reluctantly tolerated MAAF's traditional role as protector and promoter of Britain's farmers .By the mid -1980's, and following the defeat of the strike by the National Union of Mineworkers, the farming industry was disparagingly referred to within the Cabinet Office as the >green miners<.In other words, the Prime Minister's view was that the level of subsidy provided to farmers should decline, and not rise!

The satanic result was the catalyst for the emergence of a complex biochemical, known as a Misfolded Prion protein PrPsc; this evil infectious agent once it has established itself in its victim's body will silently sit and incubate waiting for an opportunity to eventually cross its victim's blood brain barrier. This Misfolded protein will then go on to wreak havoc on contact with the normally formed protein; it is able to change its shape, this starts to multiply in a chain reaction spreading throughout the brain tissue, the eventual death of its tragically innocent victim is preceded by what must be the most savage and primeval degeneration that it's possible to witness. As well as killing some 5 million cattle in the UK through BSE, it then crossed the Human species barrier and murdered my son Mark, and many, many, more innocent people.

As for the perpetrators; what satanic verses they mouthed whilst stirring their updated cauldron of death we will never know. It may have been 'Double Double Toil and trouble, round about the cauldron go. In the crushed brains and spinal cord throw, thalamus, spleen, and tonsils also, then Cool it with tainted Blood, Well done, for we shall gain a greater Profit to share with the farmers, and our meat trade. And I shall wear upon my Thatcherite brow as a reminder of my satanic power a glittering band of gold to sear the eye balls of non-believers. Infection is this brews affliction and dam all those who don't trust me.'

But tragically unlike Macbeth, Thatcherism, felt no guilt, the futile askew policy making continued unabated, and her bloody minded arrogance persisted to influence her parliamentary party.

Chapter One

"And Then There Were Two"

May 21st 1995 in the borough of Westminster. Within the confines of London's Houses of Parliament, the Witches' cat that had laid silent and unnoticed in its shadowy corner awoke at the sound of an early morning milk float humming its electric tune, the bottle jingling alarm clock that proclaimed a darker more sinister dawn.

In an adjacent mews a young colt stretched slowly and then impatiently kicked its steely hooves against a dazed box door, a light switch was thrown casting a yellow path across a nearby milk frosty farm yard floor, and ever since the molasses impregnated cattle feed had been introduced some of the milking herd were stumbling and menacingly kicking out at their parlour maids and the cat's eyes blazed yellow, two bright horizontal yellow slits in the darkness of dawn and stretching its evil torso stared hauntingly ahead, in the certain knowledge that this was the first of many that were now dead, poisoned at last by its master's updated cauldron of death. Three times the brindled cat circled and then settled slowly back into its shadowy rest, sure that it too will gain from the cauldron's flame.

For here is a Governmental pathogen more potent than any other, a legacy of incompetence; a Witches' brew so infectious that there remains to this day no cure and then, the name Steven Churchill appeared in cold blood before the cat. The first recorded death to the Human form of BSE known then as New Variant Creutzfeldt-Jakob disease, a legacy of the Tory led 1979 Margaret Thatcher's cost cutting agenda.

The following is a true story of how my late son Mark met his death through a catalogue of greed and, irresponsible Government, lies and cover up.

There was a time in our son's short life, where once normality had blown it's warm sweet breath, filled his thoughts with a clarity and vision of the future, an ability to see clearly all the colours of the rainbow, to feel the melancholy of Max Bruch's violin, concerto, and to chill out to Pink Floyd's imaginative and vibrant tones. To gain a degree at Manchester University and to look forward to a Further Degree at Sussex University.

But at the age of only 23, in September of the year 1997 all that was set to change forever.

Tuesday 19th January 2006 at almost eleven that morning a neurologist from London's medical research clinic in London's Queen Square had sat down in our small mews house in Brighton and confirmed our worst fears. That Mark, our son and brother to our two daughters, was dying of a manmade incurable disease.

A quietly spoken middle aged neurologist, dressed almost like a tailor's dummy from Savile Row, was wearing a very distinctive red and white spotted bow tie, and had seated himself opposite Mark, Eve, his mother, and myself, in our small mews lounge.

Mark sat silent and listened, the mantelpiece clock I remember thinking had stopped, as if it too were focused on that moment, we were then told the results of Mark's latest brain scan and that it had conclusively proved that Mark was a victim of variant CJD.

A single tear ran down Mark's cheek, but no facial emotions, the only words he spoke, "That sounds like a death sentence to me." Mark was as always seemingly calm and controlled. The doctor then suggested that our son may want to take part in a clinical trial in their hospital situated in London's Queens Square, and that he would take immediate steps to arrange this. I watched this Bow tied, red scarved messenger of death retrace his steps across our Mews as he made his way back to the train station. A feeling of an unwanted three dimensional emptiness flooded my thoughts.

I had recently had to bring Mark home from Ipswich where for several years he had been living, and working as a senior research engineer with British Telecom. Since 2003 Mark had become increasingly fatigued and generally unwell, and despite Mark's many visits to his general practitioner and local hospital, he was no better. In truth he thought he was suffering from Myalgic Encephalopathy (ME) an ailment that Mark had assumed to be responsible for his failing health. On 5-1-06 Eve, my wife, rang Mark's GP in Ipswich distraught and tearful, for Mark had visited us in Brighton just before Xmas and we had seen a major decline in his health, we felt distant, extremely worried and frustrated. We had had a text message from Mark saying: 'thing's ain't too good feeling v. poorly, worried about health and future'.

Finally on the 12-1-06 I visited Mark in Ipswich and took him to see his then GP, Mark had deteriorated to a level that rendered him unfit to live on his own, and so he began what must have been for him a terribly sad and demoralizing stage; having finally to lose whatever independence was left to him and return to the bosom of his family. It took me 3 days to finally prise Mark away from his lovely flat which once had formed a part of a rectory. A peaceful old house that was accessed from an unkept tree lined lane, the building flanked on one side by farmland and just a short distance from the historic town of Woodbridge in Suffolk which lay beside the river Deben. Mark's bedsit window looked out onto a church and its associated cemetery whose late medieval and part Norman façade surveyed its sleeping tenants with leaded eyes stained red green and blue, keeping a watchful eye in the Bible blackness of the night.

I remember on that visit how sad and strangely intuitive I had become about this tragic scene. I was now no longer a confident person but felt that Mark and I were being led into a lion's den with nothing but optimism and a blinded courage to protect us. I remember going for short walks whilst Mark rested, one of the symptoms of vCJD is a need to sleep and this increased with time. A short walk away from this old rectory that had been chosen by Mark specifically for its quietness I would find myself pacing the graveyard that lay adjacent to his home both tearful and terribly frightened of what lay ahead for our family.

Mark's memory was very impaired now and he needed a lot of rest. The diagnosis of vCJD finally was mentioned by his then GP, in Ipswich.

Mark rejoined his parents on the 14th January 2006 in Brighton for what was to be the last 4 months of his life. For the 2 years or more before his mother had intervened in January 2006 he had misguidingly clung to the belief that M.E had been what he needed to overcome; and why shouldn't he since his own GP in Ipswich between December 2003 and December 2005 had concluded nothing else? There were medical publications as early as 2001 describing in detail symptoms of early onset of vCJD; publications both his GP and neurologist failed to pick up on.

This neurologist based originally at Ipswich Hospital but now at the National Prion Clinic in London was not a complete stranger to our son Mark, for he had spoken to Mark in January 2004 and had explained a letter he had received from the Health protection agency. The letter had been a warning that our son had been a recipient of a tainted NHS blood transfusion in 1997 and Mark had been identified as carrying a theoretical risk of infection. Subsequently an appointment had been set up to see his then local neurologist on Monday 5th Jan 2004.

The first unforgivable mistake that the Department of Health had made was to make a mockery of all they were committed to represent i.e. protect the general public. They concealed the fact that in April 2000 one of Mark's blood donors had died of variant CJD[2] and that Mark was

---

[2] The disease named CJD short for Creutzfeldt Jakob disease had been researched by Dr Hans Gerhard Creutzfeldt [1885-1964] and neurologist Alfons Maria Jacob [1884-1931], although the term [CJD] came from German neurologist Walther Spiel Meyer [1879-1935]. The name

subsequently AT RISK. For some 4 years the Department of Health withheld this vital information on the pretence they were acting on advice from a risk assessment committee, but when I approached that committee at a later stage they denied that statement, saying it was not aimed at my son specifically. (Oh really). Specifically or non specifically this misguided decision seemingly characteristic of government decision making then and now, almost 'it's heads we vote this way tails the other, now who will spin the coin today?'.

At a much later stage they finally saw the error of their poor and irresponsible decision making after Mark's death and reversed that policy, again too little too late for our son. They were just getting on with their lives; these decision makers just don't get it do they? The responsibility for peoples' lives rests sometimes with them, which is a very frightening fact, but one that should not be taken lightly or without a great deal of thought.

On Monday 23rd January 06, Eve, myself and Mark were driven by ambulance to London, to meet with the staff who were to be involved with Mark's eventual diagnosis of new variant CJD. Mark was to join a clinical trial headed by Professor John Collinge.

The Hospital was the National Hospital for Neurology and formed part of the NHS foundation trust in Queen Square. The hospital forms part of the square and stands by a gated tree lined park of mown grass and restful benches.

Mark requested counselling after this diagnosis of variant CJD, caused by a tainted blood transfusion in 1997. During this initial meeting Mark identified two issues that were critical to him, his need to express grief, and his wish for counselling.

Mark joined the Quinacrine arm of the prion – trial in January 2006 and so started a very busy schedule. Under the direction of Professor John Collinge.

Creutzfeldt-Jakob disease finally stuck in the 1970s, after the publication of English translations of the pair's original cases.

Previously on the 31st of Dec 2003, Mark had received a letter from the Suffolk Health Protection Unit identifying Mark as having received a significant volume of blood transfusions that may carry a theoretical risk of infection, albeit this information had been suppressed, hidden from Mark by the Department of Health since April 2000! Or indeed since 1999 when one of Mark's blood donors was known to be vCJD.

It then fell to the local consultant neurologist at Ipswich Hospital NHS Trust at that time, to explain to Mark the significance of the contents of this letter, he told our son that the chances of Mark contracting vCJD were one in a million! (Oh really)

The origin of the letter was coordinated by the Transfusion Medicine Epidemiology review study started in 1997, and funded by the Department of Health. What preceded this letter was simply a catalogue of lies, cover up, deceit and incompetence. This one letter that Mark's neurologist in Ipswich who saw Mark at 10 am on Monday the 5th Jan 2004, in fact should never have been sent to him, but instead aimed at a specialist who was experienced in the field of tainted bloods and early onset of vCJD because at what was later to be our son's coroner's inquest, this neurologist was to admit at the time of seeing Mark in Jan 2004 to know very little about vCJD and its symptoms!

The question remains then why did our son not get referred to someone with experience in this field, since obviously the initial neurologist had very little? This beggar's belief!

Now where I start this tragic story is a dilemma. I would like to begin many years ago with the sun shining on his then blonde hair, this blue eyed boy with a lovely smile and perhaps more importantly always a loving and caring nature. He was a loving brother to his 2 sisters, one his elder by 3 years and one his junior by 6 years.

Our family were born in Brighton, Sussex and Eve and I leading as much a life as normal. I had always encouraged

Mark at an early age to spend time with computers knowing in the 80's it may be a good future for him and he took to computers like a duck to water, from an early stage becoming very computer literate, eventually gaining degrees both at Manchester University and later at Sussex University.

Mark was to go on to join British Telecom at Martelsham Heath near Ipswich in Suffolk in their research and development department and went on to become a senior research engineer there. He gained a very significant BT Innovation Award and a paper published in helping the aged with Alzheimer's, very ironically and cruelly strange, that Mark's final diagnosis of vCJD was an incurable disease that closely resembles this condition, a brief summary then of Mark's life before entering London's Neurological Hospital in WC1.

This chapter though should conclude with an explanation of its title.

(And then there were two) because our son Mark in 2006 was only the second person in the UK (as far as I am aware) to eventually die of Variant CJD, the human form of BSE. Or as the nation's press so eloquently put it; the human form of Mad Cow's disease as a result of a tainted NHS Blood transfusion.

And the present Tory Government in a vain attempt to perhaps mask for them what must be their annus horribilles of errors within their minions of right wing foot soldiers are attempting to rewrite history in re-naming Variant CJD as a Prion Disease, well it may be, but whatever name they wish to attach to this incurable disease I suggest they were the trigger and amplifier of this man made pathogen. The Horn review concluded that in the late 70's and early 80's changes in rendering practices produced a ten-fold increase in TSE infectivity, the feeding of MBM to young calves, a high ratio of sheep infected with Scrapie to cattle, never learning from history that by opposing nature in the way sheep breeders did in the 1700's in the UK by experimenting with in breeding in an attempt to fatten livestock by trying to modify nature's way. The process of in breeding contravened the wisdom of farmers;

it violated a sense of the natural order setting themselves in opposition to their creator by endeavouring to destroy nature, they opposed thousands of years of natural selection.

It was only when European Sheep farming gave way to the thousands of acres of Australian sheep herds, that Scrapie was reduced to a manageable size in the UK and Europe and only once reared its ugly head in good old Aussie in the early 50s and that only because of a UK import. It was contained and eradicated swiftly. It touches the same nerve that cloning does today, they are now talking animal cloning, and crop cloning, there is more madness afoot, and even crazy ideas like re-introducing a protein meat enriched animal feed back to livestock G-D; give me the strength please. And there is evidence that Scrapie has existed since the mid 1700's but its reason never really clear, one theory is that sheep because they often overgraze the land they are farmed on ingest their own faeces; Placenta, the result being the same mis-folded Prion protein that was Kuru, CJD, BSE. What is fundamentally clear is that Scrapie affected sheep were fed back to livestock, when will they ever learn?

In Darwin's Origin of Species he wrote: 'Not one man in a thousand has accuracy of eye, and judgement sufficient to become an eminent breeder', but Artificial selection was chosen against the more commonsensical natural selection Darwin spoke of, and the truth on how we should all pay heed to, Mark read, and inwardly digest his theories were trashed for greed and profit, all of these sorcerers 'setting themselves in opposition to their creator by endeavouring to destroy nature's way of progressing' in what was once a green and pleasant land.

Chapter Two

A Tragedy Unfolds

On Monday 23rd of January 2006 we arrived at the institute of neurology, in London, we that was myself, Eve and Mark were met by a member of staff who formed a part of the team associated with Mark's clinical trial. Our son was then taken to a ward shared only by a bed and side table, Eve and I were to join him later.

I can't recall exactly at what time or indeed what triggered this enormous feeling of utter despair, whilst sitting nervously in the waiting area within range of Mark's ward. I felt the need to run away from this tragedy and hide from its cold steel like truth; that our son, this lovely boy who had blessed our family with such happiness was dying of an incurable disease.

Making my way out of the waiting area I found myself one floor down sitting on some cold marble steps and weeping tears of sadness, the realization that Mark was now on death row and there was nothing I could do to save him. There are tears that are cathartic and transformative and tears that are insoluble, that day I wept the latter .I Retraced my way back to Marks ward in a silence that was drowning me ,this anechoic space challenging my very sanity ,when my senses were invaded with a tune from the production of Blood Brothers "Tell me it's not true " sang its soulful tune with a melancholy that penetrated my Fractured persona and underlined the expectation of losing my son to a Psychotically challenging ministerial Scrum ,and our family acting out this Tragedy with the Staff of a London West End Neurological Hospital ,we had complimentary tickets and front seats to both Matinee and evening performances.

On re-entering the waiting area I could hear somebody seemingly in a lot of pain, a red light was flashing outside of ward 7. A very agitated lady beckoning to staff to help the occupant of that room, who appeared to be having a stroke, some 10 minutes later and the ward was silent again. The pained patient in room 7 had died leaving only a very distressed widow to her memories, pale with shock, a lip biting, tear jerking wife who's sun had just set on life as she had known it. I got her a coffee, she said nothing. I felt empty and returned to my son's ward.

Mark wasn't there. The nurse when I enquired said he had gone for further tests with a neurophysiologist in another part of the hospital.

I sat on Mark's hospital bed, having left Eve to do whatever kept her sane, and stared numbly through the ward's hospital glass. Part of this neurological hospital ward looked down upon Great Ormond St Hospital for Children. I shuddered when I thought of those children and parents who were perhaps suffering in a similar way.

Terribly frightened and angry at the extraordinary injustice of this cyber world that we had now unwillingly entered, wanting so desperately to escape this witches' curse.

I don't remember how long I had been sitting in this trance like state, when Mark re-entered the ward in a wheelchair pushed by a hospital orderly, his face showing no emotions. Mark; just another chess piece being moved around the board, his challengers; grand masters of this game of death by design, a prerequisite of greed and insanity, thoughtless decision makers, a product perhaps of the Iron Lady's curse.

At this stage I found myself continually struggling to say the right thing to my son, trying desperately in any conversation not to upset him for if I am honest sometimes in the past, I had problems when engaging in conversation with my son, and for sure he was aware of his dad's failure to engage his brain before he spoke sometimes.

That however was truly in the past, now and before our son gets check mated by this very Infectious Prion Queen, we needed time above all time with our beautiful boy, I remember holding his hand and then thinking of a short time ago when I had visited Mark in his flat in Ipswich. He was unwell then, his apparent illness being chronic fatigue syndrome, by this time he had become too unwell to pursue a full time career with British Telecom, and did his best working part time from home.

Remembering my visit that day as if I can ever forget it, climbing the staircase and seeing Mark as he opened his flat door he engaged me with a haunting stare, and one that visits me in my darker moments. It was at this moment that I first realized there was something terribly wrong with my son, his facial expression betraying the onset of an invasion of this neuronal predator. I recall hugging him blindly and somehow desperately trying to transfer my strength and well being to him, a spiritual transfer that was in the 4th division of challenges, trying to outwit a misfolded protein that was top of the premier corrupted protein league, and he had more chance of winning the lottery every week for a year than to reverse his destiny at that stage. Nothing I or anyone else could have done then would have changed anything.

The Prion Army were on the march and winning their battle with Mark's battle scarred brain, but they were silent invaders like the black painted stealth bombers of the United States Air Force, they came with no obvious force hiding their evil path and leading us to believe that chronic fatigue syndrome was the underlying health issue with Mark. That visit was Jan 06 and had been prompted by his failing health.

Eve and I then spent two days within this department of Neurodegenerative Disease, finding out about Mark's fatal onset of Variant Creutzfeldt-Jakob disease. The staff attached to Mark's case were very thorough and thoughtful in the main. As I had mentioned earlier it was decided by Professor Collinge and his team for Mark to take part in a clinical trial, the drug that was to be used is called Quinacrine a derivative of Quinine, used during World War II, as an anti malaria drug, sourced from the bark of the cinchona tree. Quinacrine consists of very small molecules, and subsequently is able to cross the blood brain barrier easily we were to learn.

Had we known at the start of the trial in 2006 that this drug had already failed by as early as 2001 over 300 other Prion disease sufferers, would we have agreed for our son to take part? We were unaware at the time; we were clutching at straws perhaps but needed something, anything to cling on to was better than nothing.

So this; the impossible situation that Mark and his family now found themselves in, that our worst fears that Mark was vCJD had been confirmed.

A complete nightmare but every time I pinched myself, the normality of life did not return. I remember clearly at the conclusion of the first day at Queen Square's Neurological Hospital having to leave Mark in his lonely ward, god knows what he was thinking. On exiting the hospital the park gates opposite were locked as we headed away from this dreadful situation, there was something about that scene that perhaps the painter Lowry could have captured. A busy, bustling square where the famous artist of yesteryear could have cemented both the atmosphere and feeling of the two matchstick people who had just left their half extinguished matchstick son behind on a hospital bed smouldering.

Although maybe painting the scene admirably Lowry could never have drawn our shattered emotions. The refuge where our lovely son Mark Adam Buckland was staying that night, was not one he would ever had chosen. It was a temporary sanctuary for someone whose life and hopes had been taken away and that day was the saddest day of my life.

A hotel situated near the hospital had been pre-booked by the hospital for Eve and I, and was ok, I remember laying on the hotel bed that evening struggling to come to terms with the events of the day, and the confirmation of a diagnosis that had put our Mark on death row. I remember the feeling of helplessness, of frustration, anger and disbelief.

I had a strong urge to return, to the hospital to pass the locked iron gates of the park and hold Mark's hand again, instead all I could do was cry, wiping away tears of deep sadness, a waste paper bin full of soggy emotions I cried all night and I don't think I will ever stop. Looking at my watch it was 4am, couldn't sleep, the silence only occasionally disturbed by a passing car below in the street, whose occupants were oblivious to our pain. And this awful drama that lay before our family was just beginning to spread out its black carpet, inviting us to walk down its torturous path. I knew only one thing; I wanted my Mark to be well again, I remember looking across at Eve who had mercifully managed a little sleep, and thinking how lovingly protective she had been when he was younger, he was always a model of niceness.

I am hurting terribly again and unashamedly crying, I can't stop, I love you Mark and no longer believe in any God.

The second day at the neurological hospital was no better than the first, when seeing Mark I remember thinking he looked lost, he must be so tired, glancing around Mark's ward surrounded by doctors and consultants all of them eager to examine and probe Mark's battle scarred brain, this vicious mis-folded Prion army of deathly invaders were marching and relentlessly destroying our son's central nervous system and any chance of survival.

We eventually departed the hospital at around midday I remember, armed with a trial drug of Quinacrine and a prescription for more. As much as the neurological hospital is so important to the research of this manmade disease of new variant CJD, I for one was relieved to head back towards Brighton and our small mews house in a cul-de-sac where once there had been only pleasant dreams, but had now been replaced by a living breathing nightmare and was the beginning of a journey nobody would want to travel, slowly eating away your normal mental state.

I can remember that journey very clearly and recalling how my son had undergone an operation at Hope Hospital, Salford near Manchester in the year 1996, he initially from an early age had suffered from Ulcerative Colitis, a condition in all probability that was brought on by psychological bullying during his time at secondary school.

The perpetrators know who they were and they all suffered from something called Alpha Askew Syndrome, psychological bullying is inherent in our society and needs eradicating.

Mark subsequently whilst studying at University in Manchester underwent a serious operation in the form of a total Colectomy, he was under the care of a Mr Nigel Scott. That operation had seemed to be a success and Mark after convalescing returned to complete his third and final year at Manchester University

The following year in September 1997 he underwent a Proctectomy and formation of ileo j-pouch. It was then at this stage, as if Mark hadn't gone through enough, he developed evidence post surgery of intra-abdominal bleeding. A further exploratory laparotomy seemed to deal with this problem but because of further internal bleeding Mark was transferred to Hope Hospital's Intensive Care Unit. Mark was to then be transfused with approximately 40 units of blood, 22 units of red cells, 15 units of fresh frozen plasma and 3 platelet doses.

Requiring a further laparotomy and intensive care management, he eventually went on to make a good recovery and spent the next 4 weeks convalescing on the wards. But he had entered Hope Hospital with dreams that were to be shattered firstly with a blundered operation, but more importantly one of the units of blood that were supposed to save him, that he had been transfused with, went on to kill him 9 years later.

The Witches within Westminster were ultimately responsible for this tainted blood, but only seemed interested in trying to cover up their crimes with lie upon lie; a path of deceit. When John Gummer was secretary of state at MAAF he insisted that market forces play a major part in separating out what people do not want and what they know is not good for them. The common sense of the consumer should never be underestimated (MAAF 1989). What was really happening was the government's approach, avoiding new regulations, and if possible to dismantle existing regulatory controls, to further reduce public intervention and expenditure. Shortly after Thatcher came to power it was reported that (The Ministry of Agriculture wants to reduce the enthusiasm of monitoring food standards and further not to be responsible for food hygiene) 1979.

MAAF effectively with the whole hearted support of the Prime Minister adopted a policy of saying there were no risks whatsoever to human consumers and that the dead end hosts to BSE were cattle. In so far as MAAF could have been said to have had a Risk Assessment Policy. In real terms it was a policy not to assess the possible risks. What Thatcher and her sorcerer's apprentices ably assisted by, every other parliamentary party in the House of Commons lacked was common sense that intuitive instinct that separates the winners from the big time losers. And I wonder just what the wayward and askew Government of the day would say to the relatives of new variant CJD patients, all of them unwilling participants in a lottery of death from BSE infected beef products, all of these cases had the same variation (MM at codon 129 on the PRNP gene) in their genetic make-up, but we now find the more resistant markers VM and VV may well be susceptible after longer incubation periods as in Kuru.

But one such case has arisen already and so the possible protection of the other genotypes may be misleading. We were nearly into Brighton now and the realization of my son's now unavoidable decline were uppermost, in my thoughts, anything my brain was trying to decode from this tragic witches' curse was lost to the sound of the driver opening the ambulance door and spilling Mark into a now surreal and soon to be undiscovered country. A country as Shakespeare so perfectly put it from where no traveller returns.

Chapter Three

Blessed With Friends

Thursday the 26th January 2006, two days after our first visit to the neurology hospital in London, there was lots happening as you can imagine. Already the National Care Co-ordinator for the CJD Surveillance Unit in Edinburgh had made contact with our family and was subsequently able to provide an amazing amount of assistance. And today we were visited by a consultant neurologist also from the CJD Surveillance Unit in Edinburgh together with figures who were representing the national Prion Clinic in London. All went on to be important figures over the next few months; the outcome of Mark's recent spell at the neurological hospital and latterly the visit by a neurologist from Scotland was that Mark had fulfilled the diagnostic criteria as a probable case of the incurable disease of vCJD. Our whole world as our family had previously known it was now turned on its head, Eve and I made arrangements for Mark's bedroom to be converted into something larger, remembering we lived in a reasonably small mews house and Eve and I converted the garage into our bedroom for us to sleep in.

Mark had been someone who for the previous two and a half years was trying to understand why he was becoming so progressively ill, and not worrying his parents. Tragically Mark held on to his diagnosis of ME as his medical notes and his GP's diagnosis never mentioned vCJD until December 2005 despite the 3.8 year delayed warning from the Health Protection Agency in January 2004. Mark was clearly displaying symptoms of onset vCJD, and despite these facts his GP and the neurology Dept at Ipswich Hospital, failed to recognise the reason for his deterioration!

At this moment in this book I would like an opportunity to sum up how we had arrived at this point. The Witches' Brew;

the Specified Bovine Offal or SBO for short and converted to MBM (meat bone meal) both intended to increase the farmers' milk yield and the quality of beef, and reduce the feed bill. It fed cattle, sheep, dogs and cats, zoo animals; the cooked and ground up remains of other cattle is horrifying enough, as it is of course forced cannibalism, cows and sheep are vegetarian by nature. Moreover Britain was alone among European countries in feeding meat and bone meal to dairy calves, switching from milk, hay, vegetables and fish. During the first year of the BSE outbreak in 1985 when it was first recognized by MAAF'S central laboratory BSE-infected cows were themselves sent to knackeries where all of the previous safety standards had been withdrawn, the cows were rendered down, added to protein supplements then fed back to dairy herds. Naturally herbivorous cows were turned into carnivores. But eating the inadequately rendered remnants of their own species turned them into cannibals and isolated BSE outbreaks soon became an epidemic.

In short the outcome was a trigger for amplifying BSE. The first indication that human prion diseases might be transmissible through infected tissue came with the discovery of a strange disease called Kuru among the fore people of Papua, New Guinea in the 1950's. Much of the early research into the reasons this disease was prominent was by Michael Alpers, and a brilliant but eccentric researcher Carleton Gajdusek. They found as part of the practise of Endo-cannibalism, village women usually opened the bodies of their kin at tribal funeral feasts with sharp bamboo knives and stone axes. Their children sat around them as they cut open the body. The women removed the head, and fractured the skull to get at the brain. Soft brain tissue was scooped barehanded into cylinders of bamboo for cooking in the ashes of their fires. Blood and tissue undoubtedly splattered onto the children nearby. Many would leave the cadaver tissue on their hands and bodies as another element of their mourning. Kuru mainly affected women and children because the men of the tribe shunned brain in favour of muscle which they enjoyed, Kuru began with unsteadiness of gait, shakiness and lack of co-ordination. Behavioural changes followed, although dementia was unusual (making it different from sporadic CJD). Eventually the patient would become unable to move and death would follow, usually within a year of onset of symptoms. The brains of these patients showed severe damage to the cerebellum, the part of the brain which controls movement. There were also spongiform changes, characteristic of prion disease, where the brain tissue has a spongy appearance when viewed under a microscope. A further sign was the appearance of small deposits called plaques within the brain tissue.

Kuru was eventually linked to the funeral practices of the Fore people, in which it was common for the women and children to handle the body of their dead relatives. In order to test the feasibility of transmission of this incurable disease between species Gajdusek together with Alpers in August 1963 injected a Kuru brain solution taken from an 11 year-old Fore girl into a chimpanzee called Daisy, the following month a 13 year old boy, another Kuru victim had his autopsy and brain removed and a liquefied sample injected into another Chimpanzee who was given the name of George, both injections given into the left frontal cortex and within a few minutes the respondents were up and walking around normally. Some 20 months later early signs of progressive Ataxia and tremors were noticed, in May 1965 an increased abnormal behavioural change was noticed, in late July 1965 both Chimpanzees were displaying the same features as humans did in the Fore tribe when stricken with Kuru. In Oct 1965, George was gently put to death, Daisy followed in December of that year. The transmission of CJD to chimps soon followed which finally proved it was an Infectious disease. In the world of neurology it was big news, but elsewhere barely noted. This was a big mistake when it came to Thatcher's minions of advisors and scientists who didn't hesitate to promote feeding the ill rendered brain and spinal tissue back to both livestock, amplifying BSE and eventually led to vCJD crossing the human species barrier to murder many human beings. It is not known how many people will develop vCJD, however, if it is like Kuru, which has an incubation period of up to 40 years, there could be many more cases.

The Government in 1990 continually denied and played down any suggestion that this Prion protein, this misfolded TSE that had been ladled from the witches' cauldron would cross the species barrier. John Gummer on May 16th on Newsnight; his portrayal of feeding his four year old daughter a burger trying to deny that BSE posed a hazard was both pitiful and a lie. Yes of course this TSE, this Transmissible Spongiform Encephalopathy, was so infectious that it went on to cross the human species barrier and murdered a lot of innocent people, one of these was my beautiful son.

I wonder if all of the people involved with MAAF and SEAC during the Tory leadership of both Thatcher and Major and spilling over into Blair's Government can actually sleep at night, for I think it would be true to say, BSE, and its legacy of vCJD was a disaster waiting to happen. The UK authorities claimed to be protecting public health, but in reality they were only supporting agricultural markets and minimising expenditure, too little invested in scientific research. In truth it chose a path in what seemed to have zero risk but struggled to sustain that position in the light of accumulating evidence to the contrary.

I have just returned from a friend's funeral today and although I remembered this man's life, it was Mark I was shedding tears for in this small 13th century church in Patcham Village. This area was where I had spent all of my younger life, since my late parents had chosen this place to settle when they were married.

Although the Tory Government were well placed with their Black Prion Queen and set to end the game shortly, Mark still had some very good friends, and our family have a lot to thank them for over the next few months. I was astonished at their achievements in accomplishing what I can only describe as a selfless desire to guide Mark through this tragic maze. They know who they are, and at a later stage in this book with their permission, I should like to describe their dogged determination and love for Mark and our family, without which, life would have been even more unbearable.

Friday 27th January 2006, Mark's counsellor from the Prion Clinic in Queen Square came down, also an old friend of Mark's from his university days in Manchester visited, she had always maintained a close contact and seemingly was always there for him.

All the wheels were it seemed now at last being set in motion for Mark's care. Over the next few weeks an enormous input, no longer a man who had been struggling since May 2003 to understand his illness. It was only now after over two and a half years of walking in a wilderness of misdiagnosis that finally it had been revealed to Mark that he was dying of the human form of BSE, the cauldron of poisoned protein was in its final stage of destruction and all anyone could do was to be a spectator of this cursed legacy of profit and greed.

Today a letter from the CJD support network arrived, it was signed by Gillian Turner who was and still remains national co-ordinator offering support for our family and others for this devastating condition.

Mark at this stage was still able to walk with the aid of a stick and converse fairly normally, he had lost quite a lot of weight, but still had a fairly good appetite.

Some memory loss was apparent.

Today Sat 28th Jan 06, Mark still in pain with his legs. Letter to Mark's new GP now he is living with mum and dad, from the National Prion Clinic, Queen Square, London.

The letter was discussing Mark's recent admittance to the Nuffield Ward at the National Hospital, from his neurologist saying that Mark had been diagnosed to have chronic fatigue syndrome since May 2003 but started deteriorating Aug 2005, with worsening short term memory span, confusion irritability and depression. This was wrong as Mark started to deteriorate in 2003! (see medical history).

His recent MRI brain scan at The National Hospital on 6th Dec 2005 had showed a Positive Pulvinar sign. (Suggestive sign of vCJD) his neurologist at that time had waited until the

11th hour, until the barn door was within an inch of his nose before acting.

The diagnosis of Iatrogenic vCJD was discussed by Mark's counsellor, and a confirmation that Mark was to take part in a clinical Prion 1 trial with the drug Quinacrine.

I remembered how Mark had desperately struggled in trying to learn as much as he could about his previous diagnosis of Chronic Fatigue Syndrome, and here from the website he set up, Mark in his own words describes his illness:

I fell ill mid May 2003 with what seemed at the time a flu like illness. I need about five and a half hours rest a day to have some resemblance of a life. I work now part time from home – I am extremely lucky to have a very understanding employer [BT]

My main symptoms are fuzzy head/foggy head from any kind of mental activity and muscle aches if I do too much, physically. I crash if I go beyond my limits.

I use pacing to manage my life and do as much as I can.

Something else that was extremely interesting when Mark was attending therapy in 2005; he was told not to discuss it with anyone, he was told it would hamper his progress (Oh really) .The mystery deepened.

Mark from April 2003 until Dec 05 trying to progress in an illness he never had, in Sept 05 he wrote:

I've done too much physically. I went to my sister's in Exeter, not in my normal surroundings, or having my usual body protective thoughts.

On the Friday my muscles really ached. I should have stayed in bed and done very little to let my muscles recover. I spent the weekend with my sister doing enjoyable activities "and paying dearly for not resting for a few days was in a lot of intense pain, and now I can just about walk for 3 or 4 minutes without having to sit down for a break. So this is my warning to those people who are told to "dump" pacing.

I know we are all different, and that might work very well for others, but people, just be careful.

Mark spent the best part of 2005 with a CFS Blog on his own website because he believed he was suffering from CFS! Quite Why? His own general practitioner failed miserably in every way to connect his vCJD warning in Jan 2004 with the symptoms he had been so obviously displaying since May 2003 and up until Jan 2006 is beyond belief. Time and again in Mark's patient review his symptoms were constantly referred to as CFS .

From an Information sheet on variant CJD that I was given in 2006 and was published in 2001, it clearly states symptoms of variant CJD, initially anxiety, (Mark's GP's medical notes in July 2003 said he displayed anxiety).

Secondly pain in limbs, (leg pain GP's notes Sept 2005)

Unsteadiness in walking (difficulty standing GP's notes Sept 2005)

So there was a clear established link between Mark's warning in Jan 2004 that he may be at risk from vCJD, and known published symptoms displayed by Mark in his many visits to his surgery in Ipswich. And throughout this medical farce the diagnosis remained Chronic Fatigue Syndrome.

In another communication to his GP Nov 2005:

I am writing to kindly (and sheepishly) remind you about me. It's been a few weeks now since you thought it would be a good idea if I saw a neurologist regarding my legs. Are there any movements on this? My life is definitely not a bed of roses at the moment. The physical pain as well as the psychological pain my illness brings, bears no solace for me at all. What would be of some comfort to know is that the pains are due to x and y will treat the pains-or even to know for definite that there is nothing that can be done about my pain apart from painkillers. Things have really gone downhill for me I'm anxious for news.

Take care Mark Buckland.

My late son's general practitioner failed in her duty of care to identify Mark's specific symptoms, in spite of the eventual warning from the Health Protection Agency which was four years too late. Mark was surrounded by incompetence within the NHS of the highest order, shame on you, I will never forgive or indeed forget.

Wed, Dec 07, 2005, Mark after almost a year online chasing an illness he never had finally said,

"*I have given up. So during the last couple of months, I have been progressively getting worse and a couple of weeks ago I decided to quit my online reverse therapy sessions – my life was too full of pain to deal with other stuff. So that's it I am afraid, I hope my Blog has been helpful to someone out there. Mark.*"

Sat 28th Jan 06 came with a phone call from a colleague of Mark's at BT, he arranged to visit Mark at home the next day. They had previously been good friends and shared I believe a common interest in photography.

Mark's interest in photography was well known by everybody who knew him, he had a natural talent allowing him to discover beauty in even the most ordinary subjects.

As a student, Mark's talent netted him a job as a camera operator for his Uncle Van's independent Video production company in Manchester. This is of course was where Mark was at University and proved to be a valuable learning curve for Mark's photographic enthusiasm and a valuable source of income for a hard up student.

Mark could also be found cycling around the Pennines with his trusty camera whenever he had some free time on his hands.

Despite pursuing a highly successful career in IT, Mark continued to develop his talent. He had worked as a society wedding photographer, a camera operator for broadcast sporting events, an official photographer at the 1999 Labour Party conference, and went on to set up a small business selling limited editions of prints and postcards of his own work through, (mark buckland.com)

Sun 29th Jan 06. Mark's BT friend arrived in the afternoon from Ipswich, they had a lot to talk about. He was helping our family set up a broadband link primarily for Mark, who was still able at this stage to cope with computers albeit a little slower and for a shorter time.

So here we were, Mark's obvious symptoms are poor memory, and concentration, difficulty reading, and an increasing amount of unsteadiness, accompanied by some falls, he had also lost a considerable amount of weight. Mark's new GP was already referring Mark on to district nurses, with no active support at present, but they were to go on a little later to give invaluable help.

It was the early evening when Mark's friend left, having now seen at first hand Mark's deterioration and he was visibly upset.

This Sunday marked the beginning of a majorly active period for Mark, his family and good friends. Prior to the eventual discovery that Mark was vCJD both Eve and I were working, Eve had a part time job working for a local doctor's surgery, and me working as a caretaker at a local school, both employers were very understanding of our situation and allowed us to take time out to become full time carers.

Chapter Four

A Progressive Disease

Monday 30th Jan 2006, a further visit from the national care co-ordinator in Edinburgh, National CJD surveillance unit, arranging some financial assistance with everything that needed to be put into place for Mark's care package, it was a massive undertaking, and was dealt with very efficiently.

Our small shower room was to be converted into a wet room allowing the washing and hygiene of Mark who was soon to be mostly wheelchair bound and to a greater extent dependent on his carers.

It also became extremely apparent that the two small bedrooms that formed part of our house needed to be made into one to accommodate Mark's requirements for care and nursing.

At this particular stage of Mark's now rapidly progressive illness, although he could walk with the aid of a stick it soon was to become evident that he would before too long need a stair lift, all of this increasing agenda being met head on by this lassie from Scotland, the care co-ordinator Margaret Leitch.

The same day Mon 30th Jan 06, a visit from our district nurse, all of this support was of course now a very welcome and an important requirement for Mark's rapidly declining health. A suitable assessment was made for Mark's needs, I can clearly remember how painful it was when the subject of a 'Zimmer frame' was discussed, Mark now mimicking a person who was in the very winter of his mortal life.

We had noticed rapid changes in Mark's physical abilities, for instance in just over the two weeks since he had been living with us he had gone from being able to walk down stairs from his bedroom to the lounge area, to having to slide down on his bottom, no one mentioned it, just an acceptance of Mark's decline, we could not possibly have known just how much pain and trauma lay ahead.

In October 2003, the sting in the tail for the Government, the first recorded death by a Tainted NHS Blood Transfusion; Deryck Kenny (but there may well have been more that had gone undetected before and since).

In wasn't until July 1998 that the rendered cattle products such as meat and bone meal (MBM) were banned, but only from feed intended for ruminants dairy and beef herds but not for pigs and other animals and the UK continued to export long after the ban in the British Market (unbelievable isn't it.)

Banning Cannibalistic food was a very easy thing to accomplish, again the Tory Government with tongue in cheek allowing people to assume that BSE was only attributable to the feed and that by banning it there could be no other problem!

Infections have many ways of spreading including BSE. Injection, orally, animal to animal maternally; this research was ignored by the Government.

HIV as an example has a risk that it will spread maternally from mother to offspring. The same infection was taking place from mother to calf in the form of BSE, but nothing was done about it. It also had been found it could be spread by human blood transfusion by the Australians, but instead of erring on the side of caution, the government decided not to act! (Richard Lacey) expert in the field of BSE/CJD.

Mark had up until this stage, been alone in the shadow of an incurable man made disease and one that the Department of Health covered up in their so obviously flawed risk assessment policy, for the best part of four years they remained silent about his at risk status through a tainted blood transfusion. It plainly was not enough that he had been transfused in 1997 with the human form of BSE but the fact that the Department of Health kept it from him in the year 2000 when his donor died, although it was in actual fact 1999 that his donor became symptomatic of vCJD, was unforgivable, you may ask why did it matter since there is no known cure for this disease? Why indeed because in my opinion it could have made a big difference. In April 2000 when one of Mark's blood donors died of vCJD, had Mark been warned of his at risk status we may have had a much better chance of fighting this infection. In truth the incubation period was 9 years, and so in the year 2000 our son was only 6 years away from a place no one should have to go at just 32 years of age.

What is extremely challenging is this, that at the coroner's inquest into my late son's blood donor's reason for contracting vCJD, there was no mention of the important fact that he too had been a recipient of another blood transfusion several years ahead of his demise, which then leads me on to another question: Did it not occur to the relevant coroner at this inquest to explore all possible avenues of him being infected with vCJD or for the coroner was it a question that had escaped their mind?[3] Had it seemed that the obvious reason for my son's donor's death to vCJD had been through consumption of tainted beef, despite the assurances from his family that he never ate it!!!

There is another drug that was already in use then, and is still in use now to combat the very infectious Prion protein, its name Pentosan Polysulphate, this compound an extract of Beechwood shavings has proved to be beneficial in established prion diseases. Its main disadvantage is that it can't get across the blood-brain barrier, so in order for it to be effective in any way after the actual onset of clinical disease it has to be administered intraventricularly, to simplify this the drug has to be given via a procedure directly into the brain by way of a shunt, and pumped into the brain. For us it was never going to be an option because plainly the infectious agent; the prion protein was already firmly established in Mark's central nervous system in the year 2005.

However in the year 2000 when it had first been known that Mark may be incubating vCJD and before it crossed his

---

[3] My late son's vCJD donor had donated blood to how many other people before he died I wonder? That is another question that needs addressing

blood brain barrier, it is very reasonable to believe that this drug may have been very efficacious.

To simplify this again the sooner this drug is given, the better the positive results and I strongly suggest if Mark had taken Pentosan in the year 2000 (when the infection was only 2.7 years in incubation) in a tablet form, before the misfolded Prion crossed into the brain and neuronal system he may well still be alive today. Who could deny such a thing could not happen? The cover up had continued.

All these decision makers within the Government and the NHS; making the wrong judgements for our family and many others is unforgivable, for them a complete lack of lateral thinking, perhaps then they may have had a more considered view.

Has anyone ever contemplated just what the outcome would have been if I for instance, had set up a company to manufacture a food product, and that this commodity had gone on to kill a considerable amount of people. Would it have been enough for me to say in court that I had learnt by my mistakes! No of course not, the witches who included the scientists who colluded with the government were responsible for this updated cauldron of protein death and seemingly covered by a political immunity because they all walked away Scott free from an eventual no blame enquiry, perhaps aware that their one time leader, Thatcher, was a protein advocate reaffirming that fact every morning when she ate her breakfast of eggs. Yes those scientists who were paid to advise the Government on transmissible diseases such as BSE were being badgered and bullied constantly, what a wicked web they wove.

A notable example was the way Dr Harash Narang, an expert in the field of CJD and BSE was treated after he informed a House of Commons select committee in 1990 of his findings on a new variant of CJD and its link to BSE.

In short the Government tried to sabotage Dr Narang's work, his flat was broken into, his car's brakes tampered with, his work in 1993 trashed; it's reminiscent of a James Bond movie, the Government not only totally misleading the public but deliberately sabotaged science, by allowing BSE to cross the species barrier, leading to new variant CJD and murdering several hundred innocent victims, some ironically who may have voted them into power! In truth the UK public policy making was handicapped by a fundamental tension. The department responsible for dealing with BSE was the Ministry of Agriculture, Fisheries and Food, and it was expected simultaneously to promote the economic interests of farmers and the food industry whilst also protecting public health from food borne hazards. The evidence suggests that because MAFF was expected to meet two contradictory objectives it failed to meet either. MAAF was not just inflexible, but counter-productive and astonishingly reminiscent of the Witches' apprentices.

Tuesday 31st Jan 06. Visits from NHS Community Nursing, an assessment as to Mark's needs, also a visit from a representative from what was to be an important hospice for our family; the Martlets Hospice, situated in Hove.

I remember this avalanche of charged emotions that overtook me, I was now that vividly painted person whom Edward Munch had so famously portrayed in his painting of The Scream, I was crossing the bridge that separated an everyday normality to a battlefield where I faced an army of outrageous incompetence, but that was their weapon of destruction.

Revengeful, for the way it was destroying our family, I also remember a distinct feeling of mistrust, but needing all my mental and physical abilities just to cope with helping Mark survive in what was to be the culmination of a tragedy of Government errors.

Wednesday 1st Feb 06. Mark's friend from BT arrived, finalizing the installation of the broadband connection aimed amongst other things in establishing an efficient route for Mark and his very supportive band of friends to maintain contact. A very effective website was installed dedicated to this end proving to be invaluable for our family.

Today, Mark's counsellor arrives from the National Prion Clinic.

Arrangements made today for Mark to visit Martlets Hospice and Day Care.

In the afternoon an occupational therapist made a visit, and all of this time our son was now aware of the inevitable outcome of this tragedy, at just 31 years of age.

He did not deserve such a fate, for he was truly a man of worth, an individual blessed with a caring and loving character that nobody who had the good fortune to meet him would deny.

In a letter from a friend to Mark.

To an unbeliever like myself, the only response to the news of your diagnosis is to curse a malign fate and bewail the absurd unfairness of life.

I suspect that you may, in a little while be able to take a view tempered by the teachings of Buddhism and I am sure it will be beneficial, in this hard time for all of your friends and family, from the reassurance provided by this faith.

I know that I speak for both my wife and myself when I say that we have deeply admired the courage and perseverance with which you handled what you were mistakenly told was your chronic fatigue syndrome. It is supremely ironical that you should have fought so long and hard against what turns out to have been a phantom, but in no way diminishes the dignity and determination which you displayed. We recognise this and salute you.

I have written to your parents to offer them any practical help.

A letter, full of compassion which was offered in our moment of darkness, showing a profound understanding and an outstretched hand of friendship.

I am losing all of life's little niceties like smiling at a friend or neighbour, I can't force it, my relationships with anyone or anything outside of my immediate family is something I'm constantly wrestling with.

Strangely it seemed the weaker Mark got in his illness, the stronger my resolve to maximize his care and protection, for all our family the beginning of a journey that was to test our sanity and was irreconcilable.

Wednesday came and went, another night of wrestling with a galaxy of emotions and in all of this time Mark's composure remained.

Today Thursday 2nd Feb 06. Two of Mark's friends visited. Mark seemed happiest when his friends were around him and that of course was perfectly understandable, both had been at Manchester University with Mark and shared a lasting friendship.

For the first time the subject of a wheelchair was discussed since it was becoming more obvious that our son was finding walking even with a stick very difficult.

Tomorrow is Friday I remember thinking, normally for most of us a fresh transition from the working week's sameness, an opportunity to escape in your very own Tardis, and experience a journey where you can bathe in the luxury of your own dreams, whatever they may be.

Our son once shared these feelings, only to have the Thatcher/Major government assisted ably by their scientific advisors remove what promised to be a bright future for him and rob all those who loved and surrounded him of a very special person.

Friday 3rd Feb 06. Visit to National Prion Clinic, Queen Square, London.

Shortly after 8am a taxi arrived, the driver a Mr Murray, its occupants now accompanied by a wheelchair for Mark.

Eve and I had requested a meeting with Professor John Collinge, the Honorary Consultant Neurologist in the Prion Clinic.

Two hours later we arrived in Queen Square, we were met by a close friend of Mark's, they discussed the diagnosis of vCJD with Prof Collinge. At this stage Mark had been offered a tonsil biopsy as a method of confirming the disease, this was too little, too late as far as we were concerned and for Mark not an option.

Mark was warned that there was likely to be publicity about his case given its public health implications and there was likely to be considerable media interest.

After his meeting his friend then took him to a photographic exhibition, that must have been a difficult task since Mark needed to be pushed in a wheelchair.

We then had our meeting with John Collinge and had an in depth discussion on his diagnosis and the likely degree of risk associated with blood transfusion from a donor incubating vCJD.

Mark was unique as a secondary (human to human transmission) case being recognised at this stage of the disease. (Although it should have been 6 years earlier)

Professor Collinge went on to explain that it was possible that such human to human cases may exhibit phenotypic differences from primary cases of vCJD.

We discussed other experimental therapies including Pentosan Polysulphate for Mark, my consideration was that option was six years too late!

It was then arranged to meet again in a month's time.

I remember my youngest daughter being at that meeting and Eve's brother, Van.

Eventually it was time to return to Brighton, I don't remember the return journey so much as this immense feeling of sadness for Mark, the utter hopelessness, and my unwillingness to accept the inevitability of Mark's prognosis.

Just before I closed my eyes that night, the thought, why could it not have been me, my son had only just begun his lifetime's adventure, as I reached over to extinguish the bedside light, my tears betrayed the utter hopelessness and a despair that subsumed my every thought.

Sat 4th Feb 06. A Martlets Nurse to help wash Mark, Eve shopping, and friends to take Mark out to lunch.

As I mentioned before Mark was blessed with good friends, today some had known Mark since Sixth Form college and both proved invaluable to our family; an inspirational source of help and I thank them both from the bottom of my heart.

Wed 13th May 2010. Yesterday I took part in a protest march from Portcullis house to Downing Street in London.

Armed with a banner that read 'Keep Tainted Blood out of the Blood Supply', and wearing a T-shirt boldly displaying a print of my late son. Almost 3 million transfusions using donated blood are given annually in England and Wales, some of these given in cases of severe blood loss following an operation, also for genetic disorders, cancer patients, etc but less than 10% of donated blood goes toward such transfusions. Most blood transfusions are non urgent, and used routinely as a top up for patients about to undergo routine planned surgery. Despite detailed guidelines, there is evidence that a 'significant percentage of transfusions are given outside of stringent recommendations'.

I was interviewed on camera hiding my true feelings of anger and deep sadness at the total incompetence for me of Margaret Thatcher and John Major's time in office as Prime Ministers. The result of madness amongst the then MAAF (Ministry of Agriculture and Fisheries), the forced feeding of crushed brains and spinal cord to the milking herds of the UK to increase the milking yield, the cannibalistic diet of feeding ruminant to ruminant, dairy farmers referred to this feed as 'cake in the parlour'. The Tory Thatcher decision to take away safety standards within the Abattoirs! The result of these actions over 5 million cattle destroyed (the compensation package to farmers cost the taxpayer millions)! countless businesses going to the wall and the murder of many innocent victims including my son to vCJD is unforgivable, the introduction of mechanically removed meat that contained the most infectious parts of BSE cattle, that were then turned into baby food, sausages, and meat pies, introduced into school meals, and these Witches Within Westminster walked away

Scott free! No law banning animal protein in all animal feed would be enacted until 1996. This should have been enough of an incompetent disaster to bring the Conservative Government down but mysteriously it didn't, the witches' spell was still abroad.

Then in January 1994 a newspaper headline 'Mad Cow the Human Link? A sixteen year old Victoria Rimmer lay blind and mute in a hospital in Liverpool, Victoria had apparently 'lived on' beef burgers. Then the statement from John Major: "CJD is contracted for a variety of reasons. There is no evidence at all that eating infected meat is one of them. Humans do not get mad cow disease". (Oh really!) Then Gummer claimed (1998) their approach was ultra precautionary and science based, however the plain facts turned out to be misleading they did not take proper account of the implications and emerging scientific evidence.

This book is not a witch hunt although I sometimes wish it could be, we know who was responsible for this tragedy, I find it unbelievable that some people wish to give their past leader the very instigator of the amplifier of the pathogen BSE a State Funeral! Their only sentence is they have to live with these deaths on their conscience, although in reality this is perhaps too much to expect, but nevertheless it is my duty to my late son to remind them of just this, and their updated, upgraded, cauldron of Transmissable Spongiform Encapolopathy.

Shakespeare once wrote in Hamlet (What dreams may come when we have shuffled off this Mortal Coil)

If such dreams come to fruition then those responsible within the Government and its associated Health Ministries are surely doomed to a hell after death!

To a non believer like me there's not a lot I can do, if there is a god he's not at home, now no starry skies, just an empty darkness.

A brief insight into differing types of CJD.

There is thought to be four distinctive types of prion diseases.

The first is known as Fatal Familial Insomnia or FFI for short an inherited prion disease, it is an autosomal dominant mutation, which means that a child of a parent with FFI has a 50% chance of getting it too.

The second type variant, is a new form of Creutzfeldt-Jacob Disease and is almost certainly caused by exposure to BSE, a prion disease found in cattle.

The third Iatrogenic CJD, this form of CJD arises from contamination with tissue from an infected person, usually as a result of a medical procedure.

And lastly Sporadic CJD also referred to as classical CJD. I have an issue with this typecast protein disease and doubt its very existence. If a disease is known to spread by infection, then why assume that some people also get it by chance? Is it another way of cleverly suppressing the numbers of deaths to variant CJD, a governmental doctoring of victims to vCJDtrying desperately to minimise the truth on its maligned policies and the dark truth of its Witches' Cauldron. Researchers see plenty of possible alternative infectious origins for these so called 'sporadic' CJD occurrences, contamination from hospital instruments, blood transfusions from people with undiagnosed prion disease (several such cases have emerged in UK), to protein supplement pills, to the Bovine protein casing used in many pharmaceuticals, cosmetics made with cattle by products. How many people have been diagnosed with so called 'sporadic CJD' when in truth it was the infectious vCJD protein that was responsible for their demise, but looks far better for their corrupt governmental figures to further reduce the numbers who have died to mad cow –human cross over TSE.

And lastly here is a theory that I share with other victims of prion diseases. Is not Alzheimer's disease linked inextricably to CJD, this neuronal predator leaving the same damage and destruction in its wake as typical CJD invasions? But that would be much too hard to swallow for our government wouldn't it.

Chapter Five

Coming to Terms

Mon 6th Feb. The national care co-ordinator in vCJD matters from Edinburgh and Mark's counsellor from the National Prion clinic in London arrived at our house.

Both proved to be an invaluable aid in re-organising our house so that Mark's failing health requirements could be met.

I remember that day, his carer taking Mark on his first visit to Martlets Hospice in Hove, it was a short distance from our house in Brighton.

The decision to familiarize our son with this hospice was I think a considered view as part of a respite for his carers and to familiarize the staff at the Hospice and prepare them for their first case of new variant CJD.

Our family will always be grateful for the care (with one notable exception) that staff afforded him.

9th Feb 06. In a letter from Mark's new GP in Brighton to department for Work and Pensions. Describing our son's clinical findings.

Memory impairment, poor co-ordination/balance.

On Clinical Trial Drug Quinacrine.

Severe Pain lower legs, walks with stick, needs wheelchair outdoors.

Very poor balance- will get progressively worse.

CJD is a progressive neurological condition, within the coming months Mark will have increased difficulty performing daily living activities, and will need 24 hour care and supervision. He will eventually be bed bound. His condition is Terminal and life expectancy short.

Within a short space of time our family were absorbed in an intense emotional battle accepting the inevitable prognosis that our beautiful son was dying was hard enough. But knowing the cause of variant CJD was entirely a manmade disaster, is totally unforgivable, criminal, and negligent.

Guilty on all counts, the conservative government and its advisors in 1979 and for years under Thatcher, a catalogue not only of incompetence but of lies, Margaret Thatcher handed on her baton of destruction to John Major. Europe banned British beef; John Major had expressed his "astonishment" at that decision (Oh really). By then events had swung out of the control of the British Government, the sorcerers and their apprentices lost the general election (could anyone ever be surprised).

The year May 21st 1995 Steven Churchill died of Human BSE now referred to as new variant CJD.

On occasions I sit and watch a DVD that was put together by Van my brother in law, an edit of Mark both captured in his youth in celluloid and latterly on video tape when he was very ill.

Van who is my wife Eve's brother was a strong presence in our son's formative years, and owns a video production business in Manchester.

While Mark was studying for a Degree in 1994 at UMIST in Manchester, his Uncle Van, trained Mark to become a cameraman, gaining experience in this field by assisting his uncle in both still photography and movie making and editing many Bar mitzvahs and weddings etc. Photography played a very important role in our son's too short a life. As a student Mark's talent netted him a job as a camera operator for Van's independent production company. He could also be found cycling, for that was another talent he possessed, around the Pennines with his trusty camera whenever he had some free time on his hands.

Despite pursuing a highly successful career in IT, Mark continued to develop his talent. He has worked as a society wedding photographer, a camera operator for broadcast sporting events, an official photographer at the 1999 Labour

Party conference and has set up a small business selling limited edition prints and postcards of his own work through, mark buckland.com.

Just how many times I've wept for my son since his death in May 2006 is probably equivalent to the amount of times I have cursed the perpetrators of vCJD.

For those parents who have had the devastating experience of losing a son or daughter you must know how we feel.

On a day in late May 2006 as part of Mark's burial and after saying prayers I watched as his coffin was gently lowered into his final resting place. Numb with grief I made a vow to one day publish a book on this tragedy.

The sad fact is it alters your life completely, distorts your views and passions, takes you into a near vertical abyss, a black hole of lingering torture, of anger, and depression. Despite I'm sure well meant words of solace from friends and the like, there's no coming to terms, no closures, only bitterness and resentment, all that's left is the love you once held on to so dearly and an unreachable goal to see just one more time that loved one who now is cold and expressionless, to sit and hold their hand and tell them how much you loved them is all that's left.

Monday the 6th of February 2006. Lots happening today; Mark back from his first scheduled visit to hospice and his counsellor has returned to London. She is able to talk to our son more freely, Mark not feeling inhibited like perhaps he might be with his parents.

Today a friend of Mark's from Ipswich visits, she brings her guitar and then re-tunes Mark's guitar.

She is a good singer and competent guitarist who very often got together with our son who before his illness very much enjoyed his music, he had a good voice and I remember years before when he had a gig in a Brighton pub.

It was always special when Mark had friends to visit, each one bringing their own warmth and deep friendship, which unashamedly they wore on their sleeves, bringing love, laughter, and maybe a little solace into Mark's new tragic world.

I remember leaving my video camera on record whilst Mark tried to sing and play along with his friend that day, and then later when playing the recording back wishing I had not, Mark no longer able to master his instrument and visibly constrained by his rapidly moving illness, after but a short while lay his guitar down, his friend's eyes betraying her realization of our son's accelerating regression.

Finally that evening, checking out a pair of walkie talkie's; an aid for Mark if he wanted to contact his mum or dad for any reason. His mobility was restricted more and more as time went on.

Last thing to do that night was to contact a close friend of Mark's regarding dates etc. for a really special holiday for Mark and some of his close friends.

They were going to a chateau in France and this proved to be an invaluable and treasured moment in what little time Mark had left.

Tuesday 7th Feb 06. Mark let it be known that he felt 'crap this morning', he was visibly beginning to sweat more, we were told by the M.R.C. Prion clinic that it was because of the trial drug he was on, Quinacrine, which was affecting his kidneys, another symptom it gave him was to turn his skin a shade of yellow.

I noticed Mark still remained assertive, I remember thinking good on you mate but it was not to last for much longer.

The same day sitting with Mark he said, "Dad."

How I still yearn to hear his voice, I replied, "Yes son?"

In a hushed voice said, "Thanks for looking after me, Dad."

I replied, "It's my pleasure," and leaving him watching TV I went and sat in another room and cried like a baby.

What has been an extraordinarily difficult journey was always heightened by the knowledge that Mark our son was always gifted with a very caring nature and had often demonstrated his ability as a calming influence to those that chose to listen. He had once been a volunteer for Samaritans and was always a good listener.

Tues 7th Feb contd. Today Mark visited the Hospice without his counsellor, the Martlets bus reversing noisily into our village mews gobbling him up only to eject him a little while later into another new environment; a place for the sick. A strikingly modern brick built refuge, welcoming its reluctant patients through wood glazed automatic doors, to rest a while in large comfortable chairs, who made friends with their more mobile cousins the wheelchairs, and sat awkwardly, inviting another sick resident to relax and a chance to close their eyes and escape awhile from the reality of their destiny.

Mark's early experiences with adjusting to time spent within this Hospice were not without their problems, because of the nature of our son's illness, his frontal lobe and its associated memory abilities were slowly being destroyed, and any period away from very familiar surroundings were sometimes very testing for him.

A representative from the Physical Disability team arrived to discuss with us our son's immediate needs, and the subject of a stair lift, a suitable wet room, and a small wheelchair were some of the physical aids that our family needed to cope with Mark's rapidly declining health.

Mark had a visitor the same day, it was Mark's BT Line Manager from Ipswich, he presented our son with a framed certificate for winning a BT Innovation award ironically for his research on behalf of Telecare for the management and care of the elderly. It was accompanied by a DVD of that presentation in Mark's absence, and was a tearful reminder of his competence as a BT research engineer before the effects of his NHS vCJD tainted blood transfusion took over.

Wednesday 8th Feb 06. It's lunchtime, my wife has gone food shopping, and left me in charge, just had some lunch with Mark, it was followed by lots of chocolate and why not. Watching some TV but can't concentrate much on anything outside of Mark knowing as I do how critically ill he has become, at the same time not wanting to predict the future, not going there for it is too painful.

A beautiful blue sky interspersed with white and grey clouds, Mark seems not to notice instead he just stares ahead.

Wednesday went and Friday 10th Feb arrived with a press release about Mark's case appearing both in the Times and Guardian newspapers. A small article, I don't suppose many people even noticed it.

An overwhelming feeling of emptiness and despair clouded our family's daily thoughts, searching desperately for a way to come to terms with Mark's illness, as for me, seeking solace in a vodka bottle, my only escape.

Meanwhile the daily medication that our son had been prescribed, namely Quinacrine was to go on to seemingly prove totally ineffective in the treatment of vCJD. Although it may have delayed a more rapid late onset of this disease.

Today we took Mark for a relaxation therapy in Hove about 15 minutes from our home address, he seemed to enjoy his head massage.

I noticed Mark's speech was a little less slurred today, but still unable in the main to initiate a conversation.

When Mark smiled it was so calming for me, although in truth the reality of this situation was so overpowering I found it hard to breathe through this journey, likening it to Mark on a runaway bus not knowing when, or how, our son's life would be extinguished.

Mark had another visit today, an old acquaintance from Ipswich, a very kind and considerate gentleman who shared with our son an observance of the teachings of Buddhism; they had spent some quality time together in Buddhist retreats in the past in Ipswich.

Despite Mark's rapidly declining health he at this stage at least retained a healthy appetite and as far as tea was concerned Earl Grey tea was at the top of his list.

Sat 11th Feb. Mark out with a good friend today, a bosom pal, they had both attended the same V1 Form college and shared many formative early experiences including if I remember playing Dungeons all night, an internet game in the early 90's.

Despite the risk of repeating myself I have nothing but the greatest respect for Mark's friends who selflessly helped Mark through this tragic period of his illness.

And along with others were all a blessing to our family.

As for Mark he sometimes watched TV and I remember our son doing various activities, at this early stage still able to use computer, and his mobile phone, with noticeable signs of slowing down nevertheless a life force we were happy to see.

One of the many side effects of our trauma, and this still lives with me, is an inability to listen to music, without developing an enormous sense of sadness, a musical link to my suppressed emotions regarding my son and my undying love for him.

Today the sun is shining on our small mews house nestling as it does between the main A23 and the London to Brighton railway into Brighton, and is for the most part clogged with what seems an unending trail of carbon spouting gas guzzling factory moulded choose your own colour and make vehicles that often project their owners perception of how they wish to promenade, they encasing their occupants in a bubble of a 5 geared, leather seated, mile eaters, their installed CD's reducing the enthusiasm for dialogue, chilling to the sound of Michael Buble, or conversely imagining you were at that live gig with Take That is a distraction from the boringly lengthy bumper to bumper experience that's part of getting to your destination as you near Brighton, especially at weekends.

In a Westerly direction we were able to idly watch the main London to Brighton Railway traffic, a continuous cacophony of people carriers ungrudgingly displaying their owner's liveries, fulfilling a mode of transport for city workers and tourist traffic alike.

Opposite our Mews entrance in complete contrast to our recently built house, a row of Victorian cottages whose feathery Grey slated roofs almost magically turned black when it decided to rain, Victorian slate, Victorian Façade a reminder of our heritage.

So this a tale so strong in its sadness you can almost taste the burnt embers of the witches' fire on your smouldering lips, their cauldron still warm to the touch. Its contents so infectious it is resistant to bleach, alcohol, or radiation and autoclaving. When doctors perform autopsies on patients who have died of Creutzfeldt-Jakob Disease (CJD) they use chain mail gloves, these are worn under rubber gloves to prevent cuts. Wearing helmets with visors the instruments used for autopsy cannot ever be used again.

Saturday evening, 11th Feb, watching TV, with Eve, one eye on the clock, Mark out with his friend and I'm concerned that he is ok, I answer my own question and realize it's because he is so ill I have these psychological panic attacks and worry unnecessarily about him. My brother in law Van always has reminded me of this fact and to be honest I think my late father was the same and maybe I handed it down to my son, a genetic relay of excessive concern which can be internalized and very stressful.

One eye closed and the doorbell heralds my son's return, I thank his friend and as his car exits our mews I notice Mark looks very tired, but not totally surprised as one of the underlying symptoms throughout his illness is a need to rest and sleep which is characteristic in vCJD.

Last thing I remember doing that day was reading an article in the Guardian, the report that the Government had set aside £30 million for vCJD cases, the report went on to say the Solicitors handling the case on behalf of the victims had been extortionate with their fees, aligning their behaviour to vultures after the lion had his fill.

Mark was on his computer whilst I read the Guardian, that night I remember thinking thank god he still understands networking, his memory is declining, it's at this stage that his short term memory is failing, his frontal lobe is suffering from the witches' brew that's converting his normal protein to a mis-folded version . The illness was incurable then in 2006 just as it is now as I sit and write this tragic story in 2011.

From time to time in my mind's eye I see London's Neurological Hospital where Mark is undergoing his Prion Trial, the park gates that adjoin the hospital are always seemingly locked, contrasting with the hospital's entrance always seemingly open, and mutedly welcoming those desperately unlucky mortals who neurologically have been dealt the cruellest path to travel.

We needed a Tardis, our own time machine to whisk us away from the reality of our son's fragility and the certainty that we would shortly have to say goodbye.

My dreams were so real, a reoccurring assortment of memories of my son in his younger days. A picnic in a lush green park, a beautiful blond haired boy with a happy disposition and a magic smile and just for that moment I could be happy again, and maybe kick a football around.

In the bath mirror I noticed I am gaining weight, I of course know why it's the vodka or whatever alcohol I needed to reduce the searing inescapable knowledge that I went to bed with, and woke up to, that I was losing my son to the government's blind stupidity and a ministry that put greed before anything else.

How many Purdey shotguns or thoroughbred horses have been paid for, how many second homes purchased, how many moated castles obtained to endorse their sense of material achievement by the profits within the meat, food and agriculture industry I often wonder, and ministers, whose only concerns were profit firmly believing nature could be modified because they knew better.

I have never been well off and used to be quite happy with my lot, an average guy with an average job not pretending to be any more important than the next person.

As a matter of fact during my youth and armed with nothing else but dogged determination in anything I wanted to achieve, regularly rode top class racehorses from two horse racing yards in Lewes, Sussex. Tom Gates was one trainer and later Mick Masson, the trainer and head lad never trying to alter the animal feed relying instead on recipes handed down from generation to generation, hay, oats, and a bran mash, more than enough to keep their animals feisty and win races. What better recommendation for using this feed when Gordon Smyth, another notable Lewes based trainer won The Derby in 1966 with (Charlottown). I also discovered that our equine friends refused to have anything to do with meat bone meal, obviously they benefit from a higher intellect than those individuals that introduced specified bovine offal as a cheap substitute to hay oats etc. I was the type to accept and be content to beat for the shoot, they on the other hand wanting their own stand and peg and a best London gun.

It was not necessary to try and play at god, but just to accept what millions of years of evolution had taught us to accept, nature's answer to survival, because it has already been worked out! We have been farming cows for over 8000 years. Then in an attempt to increase yields and maximize profits the Government and their associated scientists amplified a pathogen so infective it went on to murder at first animals then the human species. People should never forget exactly what the Tory Party have been guilty of and remarkably they are still in power! (How short are people's memories) You may say well all of the original cabinet members are no longer in power, that's not true either, but more than that it's the stubborn askew party philosophy, the insane policy making, like Martin Luther King I also have a dream and it is this, at all times think clearly and please remember your responsibility to your fellow men. All parliamentary parties share a huge responsibility to those that have elected them to power, be sure you are worthy of that often misplaced trust.

Sun 12th Feb 06: Sleepy Sunday in our sleepy mews, two further friends visiting Mark from Manchester, old friends, it was somehow sad but very sweet to see the two girls supporting Mark as an aid to his obvious decline in the ability to support himself.

Sunday came and went all of the time our family with a low mood and heavy heart, but needing strength to try and support our dear son throughout this dark nightmare of a journey we were forced to take.

Monday 13th Feb 2006: A bad day for Eve and I, we had a terrible row, not entirely surprising I suppose, both living a nightmare scenario punch drunk from every sling and arrow that this mis-folded Prion protein was developing within Mark's central nervous system.

Forget the modern fictional heroes Batman, Superman, Ironman etc that's TV, this was a reality show without a hint of a good ending, nowhere to go, just an acceptance of how cruel life can be, but not wanting to surrender, only to fight for our son doggedly and not give way to the obviously impending defeat, I sometimes wonder if the late Walt Disney's portrayal of his film The Sorcerer's Apprentice should not have carried a darker more sinister and meaningful message, one that tragically MAAF and its associated scientist chose to disregard during the Tory years 79-97, instead all the while like ostriches buried their many heads in the sands of deceit, time and time again.

I've often tried to seek moderation in Rudyard Kipling's Poem 'IF' since Mark's illness, trying, wanting to be a stronger person than I am, finding it impossible to reconcile our son's hopeless predicament only revengeful at what was irreversible, a no win situation for our family, a station platform, a train without a reverse gear, no turntable, no brakes, and the certain knowledge of shortly losing a part of our life that was irreplaceable.

Chapter Six

The Tory Carousel

It would be remiss of me I suppose, not to at this point to acknowledge my own failings during Mark's illness, indeed as I attempt to write this book my weaknesses cling hauntingly to me, triggered as they were by the man who wore the red scarf and matching bow tie, the messenger of death from the national prion clinic.

Although my wife Eve and I and our two daughters together with the invaluable contributions from Mark's good friends were all very focused on doing their best to ensure what time Mark had left was quality, this nightmare for me only eased by reaching to the back of a cupboard where I had perhaps hidden a bottle of vodka. It could have been any type of alcohol but I soon learnt vodka was pretty well odourless, and then momentarily I could hide from the dark Darth Vader like truth.

In the rare moments when I had the time to reflect on our dear son's death sentence, I imagined what I would like to say to Margaret Thatcher and her successor John Major and their attachment of sorcerer's apprentices namely MAAF and SEAC.[4] I so desperately wanted to take the pain from Mark's body. I later re-named MAAF as meaning 'Misleadingly Askew and Farcical'. SEAC was a non starter if only because some of its board members may have had financial interests within government and industry.

Mark remained until the very end an inspirational figure; never complaining but it seemed had accepted the inevitability of someone else's stupidity.

I on the other hand cannot accept the outrageously divisive cover up and lies that continued within the Conservative

---

[4] SEAC (Spongiform Encephalopathy advisory committee.)

Government, in the BSE crisis, and its subsequent crossover to the human species resulting in vCJD and the murders of several hundred individuals whose only wish was to enjoy a normal life span.

And the sentence for these witches and their updated cauldron of death; simply nothing! Furthermore in the year 2013 people are still dying of new variant CJD and BSE is currently still here in the UK, yes really do your own research and you will find the truth. Currently one poor soul in Brighton is vCJD (Sept 2013).

But strangely it's never headlined, the cover up continues, may I suggest that perhaps the news media circus as they were in the BSE crisis (with a few exceptions) are firmly in the silk pockets of governmental ministers whose only goal is to continue to suppress the for them embarrassing reality that the horror of their legacy continues unabated and there is absolutely nothing they can do about it.

The carousel of the Tory regime continues to revolve unhindered, suppressing the truth from the general public, their trusty mounts blinkered, not for the first time, intent only on winning their Grand National Lottery and another chance to continue ruling the working class. Furthermore, New Labour attacked the Tories – not for the cover-up, not for putting millions of lives at risk, not for murdering almost 5 million cattle not for the deaths of nearly 200 innocent people, but for the incompetence in defending the profits of the British Beef Industry!! They have all missed the one issue we vote, as a nation for a party to guide us through this maze of often difficult decision making, in the vain hope that somehow these civil servants, these educated public school figures, have the natural born talent to lead in a just and god like manner, the clear answer is they do not, it's very sad that above all else, that before people's health and welfare, before anything, money and financial gain is uppermost in their agenda and that needs addressing!!

And what fences lay before them, the Tories, whip in hand, and a tally ho blunder their way around intent only on entering the winner's enclosure at any cost and making a profit regardless of the consequences.

How often I wished I could calm my mind and dispel those troubles that hauntingly embrace me.

In the darkness and cold silence of night I hear no calming voices, my thoughts and eyes drawn hypnotically only to a wooden coffin whose outstretched arms welcomed my son to his final subterranean resting place.

Black gowned ministers doing their best to calm the chief mourners to lay their fears to rest.

They speak in their address of what they knew of his all too short a life before he was toppled from his trembling perch, when greed and evil overtook his expectations of a normal life and a chance to grow old gracefully.

It's now October 2011, our youngest daughter just married, and I really need to start writing again.

Time again to enter my very own time machine and travel back to relive my late son's last few months, to try and describe the horrors of this a family tragedy, a catalogue of tears and anger, of disbelief in the sheer stupidity of the perpetrators that caused him to leave us both heartbroken and I believe changed people.

In my mind's eye it's February 2006 again (how that time has flown) Mark's friend a former university colleague who had shared a house in Manchester with him and others visited, and together with other friends took Mark to lunch.

The same day in February 2006, in the evening of that day, we had a visit from our minister, Rabbi Efune, who at that time was Rabbi to our local Synagogue, a good friend, and had previously married my eldest daughter.

Rabbi Efune had always exhibited a very calming influence and has recently in 2011 married our youngest daughter, a good man and together with his family are truly people of worth.

Although a wonderful wedding in September of this year, my son Mark should have been there, we all missed him terribly that day.

I remember around February 2006 our newly installed broadband internet going wrong, but in spite of all this Sh----t, Mark remains calm (a lesson to us all). He had a god given quiet confidence that I sadly lacked and still do.

Tomorrow we meet Mark's girlfriend's parents, we had arranged lunch at the Grand Hotel in Brighton, Mark and his girlfriend on a separate table a few yards away, out of the corner of my eye I watched my beautiful son holding hands with a girl whom I believed he was very much in love with, profoundly sad I remember thinking that such a loving relationship was doomed to founder on the jagged rocks of man's unthinking inhumanity to man, Mark only just able to hold a thread of conversation.

I survived on a diet of red wine, and a sense of the inevitable reality of my son's tragic destiny. All I ever wanted for my son was coldly stolen from under my feet with the lame excuse (we have learnt from our mistakes) where in reality the real mistake was that these incompetent decision makers were ever born!

You know I was quite happy at one time in spending time in physically exercising as part of a lifestyle, to walk the foothills of Sussex, but not to scale at least mentally the bloody Himalayas except perhaps I may have grabbed a prayer shawl for my son who in the Autumn of his so short a life had chosen Buddhism as his firm belief in what a true and meaningful life pattern should be.

There is no greater or deeper love, no pain so hard to bear, than for your children when their life is threatened. Our family hurt so bad you can almost smell it.

I'm putting on weight I think it is called 'comfort eating'.

Today we took ourselves off to our local hospice called the Martlets, in Hove it was Mark's second visit to what was to be our son's refuge from a sometimes insane world.

Wednesday 15th February 2006: Case Conference Day: Too little too late for Mark, everyone involved now with his care realizing that time was of the essence.

A note from his new G P in Brighton to the team that was being set up for his care.

Mr Buckland is a young man with vCJD, his life expectancy is poor, his condition is progressively deteriorating.
Please can he have an urgent assessment.

I have to say that the care that was put in place from mid-January 2006 until his body finally gave up to this evil tainted NHS blood transfusion was in my view a very competent, pro-active and sympathetic one, and a complete reversal of the disgustingly incompetent direction firstly under the Tory Governmental Parliamentary Parties led by Thatcher and eventually Major, who went about their decision making prior to and during the BSE and CJD crisis in a continuing blind and irresponsible fashion, with seriously flawed decisions, and I suggest totally maligned dialogue that led eventually to the defeat of M Thatcher's puppet Mr John Major, and beyond into Mr Blair's Health Protection Authority equally life risk taking committees who decided in April 2000 after learning from the blood transfusion authorities that as a result of a tainted blood transfusion in Sept 1997 that my son Mark was at risk of the incurable disease vCJD deliberately concealing the facts from him instead preferring to say nothing, hoping it would go away, gambling that perhaps the worst scenario would never happen, gambling with my late son's destiny in a way you might when playing Russian Roulette except the gun was pointing at my son's head not theirs!

If as in the case of life impacting decisions one has to err on one side or another, then to be open, and truthful and base that decision on the worst possible scenario to any right minded individual has to be the only decision.

To hide the facts from Mark and his family for so long was so completely wrong it's not only incompetence personified but in law sue able! More anon.

It's now Nov 2011 and the Tory carousel continues to revolve although for me and others it has lost its bright fairground attraction a long time ago, no longer a radiant colour of gold, but exhibits a very tired and tarnished look of unpolished brass, the spectacle of gallant white thoroughbreds galloping into battle intent only on bringing honour and victory, economic stability, and believably committed ministers, who only wish to bring a truth and honesty to the table, has sadly been replaced by ageing equines, tawdry, and irresponsible, whose only objective to continue with the Iron Lady's tradition of a feudal tyranny and a wish not to dump their holy grail of profit before people, into deep dark ditches. Unwilling to believe the probability that like the BSE tainted and infected cattle they were forced to burn and then bury, won't come back to haunt them. So perhaps those ministers who were making these very questionable policies within government during the dark times of the BSE crisis will look up during their Yuletide Feast and reflect on the outcome of their floored decisions and perhaps raise their glasses to the ghosts of Xmas past, and the tears in the eyes of those families who were betrayed by them.

As well as trying to write the true story of my late son's demise, a task that I have found a difficult and emotional one, I have together with other vCJD affected relatives tried to make a difference within our NHS Blood Transfusion Service.

This should I thought at first be a fairly straightforward task since it has been admitted by our government that it was because of a BSE tainted blood transfusion in Sept 1997 that our son died of Variant CJD.

It's been 14 years since that tragic error, and 12 years since anything has been introduced within the NHS to prevent anything like this happening again.

In the late 90's a procedure called Leucoreduction was put in place designed to minimize the infectivity of transmissible spongiform Encapolopathy from blood. It was found to be only 42% effective at best and not sufficient enough to remove all blood borne TSE infectivity, there was and still remains a necessity to remove non-cell associated infectivity! In 2006 I was told by a lead within the UK Blood Service that it is a very expensive process to filtrate units of blood but wait a moment, why? Is it necessary to do this in the first place (is it not because of Governmental errors!) 14 years have passed since any attempt at a clinical reduction of infectivity in the blood transfusion service was put in place by the government, shame on you, just how many more victims of tainted blood transfusions must there be before you act?

On Friday the 1st April 2011 in the House of Commons, the present Government blocked the Contaminated Bloods Bill as in October that same year. The purpose of the Bill is to provide support for people who have been infected with certain diseases as a result of receiving contaminated blood and blood products supplied by the National Health Service, and so it continues, and always will until they stop ignoring advice from their own advisory committees.

And guess what, there is such a device available, in the case of vCJD, a scientifically proven Prion capture filter, thank the lord above you may say, only one problem, our Government will not adopt it, preferring instead to give it lip service only and continue to gamble with the publics' lives, expressing a wish to continue in their denial of a requirement for such an important issue as the safety of the UK's blood transfusion system.

My son was only one of many that have died as a result of exposure of tainted blood in the UK Transfusion Service, there are many, many more haemophiliacs who have been transfused with HIV, Hepatitis, vCJD, etc.

Ok you may say so consider this, since the NHS Blood Service could be considered a can of worms. In July 2005 around 100 blood donors were told that they may have a greater chance of carrying the vCJD agent as compared with the general public as their blood had been donated to 3 people who had since died of vCJD.

As a precautionary measure the donors were told not to donate blood, tissue or organs! For me this is nowhere good enough.

When I traced my late son's donor I had assumed that a transcript of his coroner's inquest would give me an indication of how he had contracted vCJD.

The coroner's conclusion was death by vCJD probably by eating tainted beef!

Not necessarily true; first of all it was pointed out to the inquest that the victim never ate beef.

However the verdict had never taken into account that approximately ten years before his death to vCJD he was involved in a serious car crash and required a blood transfusion!! Subsequently he had been a blood donor, the equation would seem to fit exactly, the question is how many more people have died and not had the benefit of an associated autopsy to detect a Prion disease traceable by a simple swab test of their tonsils. Or indeed a blood test which I understand has now been developed by the MRC Prion clinic but that the Government has decided not to fund? I can only surmise that if carried forward litigation would destroy some back benchers, Government Ministers and members of that elite club the House of Lords because the test may prove a lot of people positive!

Because unless the haematology unit of the UK can guarantee traceability of every blood donation to be free of Prion disease, and as far as I am aware no absolute guarantee can be given, then we all have to wait with baited breath for the eventual outcome.

What our government has put in place is the following, I hope you are all listening very carefully. Since 1998 when Leucoreduction was first introduced is this, the tracing of certain people who can be identified as 'at risk' of vCJD because of blood transfusion (e.g. from a donor who later developed vCJD) in reality this did not happen. In 2005 this same measure extended to include some people who have donated blood to patients who later went on to develop vCJD. Something like 2 million blood donations are collected every year by the UK, and in excess of half a million patients receive transfusions annually.

Full implementation of a near 100% blood filtration within the UK would only cost one pound per person, FACT.

On every unit of blood that is issued within the NHS Blood Service there is a Government health warning stating there may be a risk of contamination of prions that may establish vCJD within its recipient is not even funny it's a get out clause.

Chapter Seven

The Writing on Our Wall

Feb 2006: Mark's Case conference day in Brighton was getting painfully more legible day by day, all supplies of rose coloured glasses had been withdrawn from our family's hurting bodies, painfully tiptoeing through this minefield of a god forsaken space, just take a look at us now, hopeful of a reprieve but knowing this can never be the case, any hopes of optimism in this cul-de-sac of death are dwarfed by an incurable and untouchable Mis-folded prion protein.

My wife and youngest daughter attended a Brighton Conference designed to address Mark's clinical and social needs, I stayed at home with Mark, he slept for most of the time, an accelerating symptom of this disease.

I drank a glass of red wine, made sandwiches and a cup of Mark's favourite tea (Earl Grey).

I remember sitting down and writing a letter to Professor Collinge asking him for any medical notes history from the year 2004 onwards regarding my son's yawningly late warning from the Health Protection Authority.

Eve and Raquel arrive back home.

Feb 16th: Woke up early hours, and tried to imagine what life was going to be like without Mark, couldn't go there, too painful.

A delivery of a new wheelchair today, we placed this chair by the lounge window which overlooked our Mews, we hoped this would be a distraction for Mark during daylight hours.

A special assessment by a social worker attached to Mark's case saying our son was diagnosed with chronic fatigue syndrome. Only recently diagnosed with probable Iatrogenic variant CJD IN Jan 2006. He has a poor prognosis and now under the care of National Prion Centre, London.

Mark had a bad fall in the middle of night when he went to go to the toilet, chose the wrong direction in his bedroom to exit and crashed.

I can very clearly remember when sitting in Mark's bedroom one day and painfully searching for answers to some questions he was asking, one of these questions was can I be cured dad? In a flash I chose to lie to my beautiful son, assuring him that his medication would eventually prove to be successful, the look of relief on his pained face will never leave me until I too enter my final resting place, and perhaps meet up with him once again.

Strangely although it must have been a fairly painful experience falling he never complained about the distress it may have caused him.

His Mental Health.

Cognition and dementia including orientation and memory loss.

Depression, reactions to loss/emotional difficulties, as a result of his diagnosis, Mark is showing signs of short term memory loss and confusion, he is also reported to be presenting with irritability and depression.

He is receiving counselling support from (National Prion Centre) and is also linked in with counselling service at the Martlets Hospice.

Recent neuropsychological report (dated 24th Jan 05) indicated that Mark was orientated to person place and time, and was able to discuss recent personal and public events, however this was inconsistent with his performance tests on verbal and visual memory as these were very poor. His scores have reflected a severe and quite generalised degree of cognitive dysfunction. Mark reports to be feeling low in mood and appeared to give up easily on difficult tasks frequently giving 'I don't know' answers. Despite the memory loss and cognitive impairment, he appeared aware of the implications of his diagnosis and wishes to be actively involved in all decision making regarding his medical nursing and social care.

Self care & Physical Well Being

Personal hygiene: washing/bathing/toileting/incontinence/grooming /dressing/oral/foot/skin care

Mobility/Pain/Sleeping patterns

Mark is managing independently with his personal care routine in the morning, he also dresses independently but admits that these tasks do take a little longer to complete is currently being supported by 2 carers from Martletts at home with showering every other day, Mark admits to finding this difficult as he is used to showering daily. The bathroom is currently not meeting Mark's needs as it contains only a shower cubicle - is awaiting an adaptations assessment via Martlets OT dept for level access shower area. Mark has requested male carers to support him but has accepted that this may not be possible.

Mark is currently mobilising using a walking stick.

He has poor balance and unable to use the stairs independently. Requiring 2 carers at all times has wheelchair but waiting for a more appropriate one as the one he has is compromised by restrictions in room sizes.

Also has 3 Zimmer frames one on each of the floors suffering still from severe leg pain.

Mark suffering as if all that is going on isn't enough from continual nightmares!

Mark now linked with the National CJD unit in Edinburgh and they are heavily involved in the care planning.

And all of this caused by one unit of tainted blood from our very own NHS Transfusion Service. Can't you now see why I need to make a difference!!!!!!!

The present Government under Cameron however is seemingly not concerned with addressing the situation and avoiding, as far as possible any intervention in the obviously flawed NHS Blood Transfusion Service preferring to do nothing, but with tongue in cheek gamble with other peoples' lives and wait until others die of tainted bloods, gambling heavily presumably on their own scientific advice (I sincerely hope for their sakes this time they are right). For they failed miserably last time!!!

Feb 2006 continued: There's rumours that Stannah the chair lift company will be arriving shortly to measure for a stair lift, one of the many items needed to maximize Mark's care.

Followed Mark upstairs today and he asked me this question, "Dad how long have I been staying here?"

I replied, "About a month," again a strong reminder of how devastatingly this unmerciful and invasive disease was destroying his frontal lobe and short term memory.

Feb 17th: Collected Mark from his friend's flat where he had been spending a night away from his parents, a peaceful wrought iron, gated mews on the waterfront in Brighton. He appeared fine and I was comforted by his friend's warm caring ways, and I smiled inwardly at any sarcasm that Mark directed at me; it was his way of correcting any of his dad's waywardness.

Life in our Brighton mews was now very rapidly getting busier day by day.

A therapist provided by the NHS, their job to assess Mark's increasing needs, lots of mail arriving needing urgent replies, an innumerable amount of phone calls both night and day, life was now underlined, important, prognosis poor, life had now switched to the fast lane, and in the middle of all of this a need to meet Mark's requirements there remained a slowly fading but serene and oh so lovable Mark as ever most times smiling that smile, that expression of loveliness that only he could achieve.

I remember asking Mark did he feel that the drug that had been prescribed to him by the MRC Prion Clinic as part of his clinical trial namely Quinacrine was making any noticeable difference, his reply short and to the point as ever, "No," he replied in a sad and reflective response.

Sat 18th Feb: It's 2.45 in the morning with everybody asleep except me, just taken another 2 Paracetamol the only way I knew how to get some sleep then, my head so full of issues concerning my son's welfare, but very few answers.

Saturday came and went and in between my eldest daughter visited with our grandchildren and her husband, they had travelled up from Exeter where their Edwardian house stood a short distance from the city centre. On reflection living such a long way from Brighton must have been enormously challenging for her as she was very mindful of our dear son's fairly hopeless prognosis by know.

Met my eldest daughter and her two boys from the station, she looked tired I noted, then dropped them off at a Brighton hotel intending to collect them a little later.

My daughters were good with Mark, and my grandchildren of course acting normally, my only wish at that time was an overwhelming desire to see life back as normal. My son in law maybe finding our situation just as difficult being involved in a potentially impending family loss and all that goes with that desperately difficult maze we tried to lovingly help steer Mark through.

Sunday 19th Feb: Amongst other activities that day we joined Mark's friends who had thoughtfully taken him for a pub lunch in Ditchling, a small village just outside of Brighton.

The Bull Inn a popular watering hole, and I remember acted as a meeting place for Sunday club runs with a cycling club that I once belonged to The Sussex Nomads.

I can remember that day from some notes I had taken at that time hoping then to one day commit as many memories of 2006 as possible to a book thinking perhaps it would be important somehow to someone.

Earlier on over that weekend Mark's friends in their committed and unselfish way had volunteered to move all of Mark's belongings from Ipswich to Brighton, they fulfilled that commitment and Eve and myself helping with the storage of our son's belongings in a unit within 200 yards of our town house. Thanks guys.

I've no idea even to this day what was going through Mark's scarred mind at that time. Perhaps it's better that I didn't.

We all later discussed holidays for Mark and friends.

I felt I was imposing in the lounge bar where Mark gathered with close friends so I secreted myself into the public bar and sat next to a very attractive log fire, sipped my pint of please help me to forget the reality of all of this nightmare alcohol, and allowed Mark and his friends free rein on their plans for some special time together. Mark's life span now severely shortened, mimicking perhaps an extraordinary fast time lapse sequence, 40 years in just 4 months that's Ok I suppose if you are not Mark but a bit unfair if you are.

It was I found difficult to sit and be a spectator of normality, other people with a natural enthusiasm for life's little pleasures but after all it's what I had done until very recently. It's like some monster robot had pulled me over to the side of life's highway and directed me into the devil's own layby and told me to wind my window down to watch life as it went by and then let my tyres down. How the hell in god's name can we progress anywhere now?

My son as the song goes was the wind beneath our wings, a shining example of how we should all parade in life's green and pleasant land except, but sometimes life isn't pleasant, and the green turned a very different colour for Mark, it was tainted blood red.

Monday 20th Feb 06: Mark is collected from home and driven to the National Hospital for Neurology in London to meet with the staff in the Prion Clinic and further tests, his girlfriend was to be there and that would be of great comfort to him.

Tues 21st Feb 06: Whilst Mark was still in London, Eve and I were frantically moving furniture etc around our house to enable our son's bedroom to be extended.

Visited daughter and grandchildren in their hotel and then had some lunch with them.

Found some time to write a letter to Prince Charles describing briefly our son's predicament and of course the steps leading to this tragedy, knowing of course his enthusiasm for organic farming and realizing this cursed legacy of feeding infectious material to Bovines was not on his agenda I was hopeful of a favourable response. And indeed Mark later received a very understanding and sympathetic letter from Prince Charles, which we still have to this day.

Wed 22nd Feb 06: Mark back home now, but not for too long, another madly busy day 11.30 AM Mark's occupational therapist arrives, collected daughter and kids as an arrangement had been made for a photo shoot of the family at 12.30 that day. This was to be the very last time we as a family were to have a formal picture taken with Mark.

Later Mark went to dine out at a favourite vegetarian restaurant of his in Brighton, and I was to collect his party in the evening and I remember it was an awful wind swept and rainy ending to that day.

Thurs 23rd Feb 06: A very exciting and pleasant few days were to begin today, for Mark and his many friends, they were flying to France, a trip organised by two of our son's old school chums. A chateau owned at the time I believe by a parent whose enormously kind gesture had made life just at that moment a special place where he could say goodbye to every one of those dear people who surrounded him in his time of need.

My youngest daughter and Eve's brother Van accompanied if I remember about 12 or more, Van contributed a DVD at a later stage as he filmed various parts of their time spent together, all sharing a friendship and love they had for Mark.

On that same day Eve and I went to London to meet with Mark's counsellor at the MRC Prion Unit in Queen Square, I remember, in truth I hated this place but only because of its association with Mark's progressive disease, as I gazed upon Queen Square once more that day, from what was then a very small café at one end of the square, the scene mirrored our feelings at that time bleak, forlorn, devoid of any optimism I don't remember exactly what was discussed at our meeting, an opportunity to catch up with Mark's progress (there was never going to be an improvement) to get up to speed as the saying goes, it could also have been to discuss our need for counselling. The whole plan at this stage though, was to maximise what limited life expectations Mark had.

We had booked a hotel off Oxford Street near to Marble Arch because geographically it was close to the hospital where Mark was undergoing his clinical trial in Queen Square.

That evening we visited London's theatre land, the Queens Theatre in the West End was our venue and we watched Les Miserables, I cried quite a bit throughout that performance, some scenes having an overwhelmingly strong association with our predicament.

The hotel was rubbish, we complained as you do, the room got upgraded, but not our lives, they remained a very poor 2 star existence.

The following day saw Eve and I having lunch at a restaurant next to the synagogue where Eve and I were married in Jan 1970 in Heneage Lane, London, the building dating back to 1701. The chicken soup and Kneidels were to die for Oye Vay.

Finishing eventually that day with a trip to Oxford St as you do, and all of these things in truth distractions from the reality of our beautiful son's devastating situation and the immense pain we knew as a family we were all going through.

Fri 24th Feb: Early Morning. Lying on a London Quilt in Granville Place WC2 contemplating what the day ahead may bring, happy only in the certain knowledge that our dear son was now surrounded by a loving circle of friends within a chateaux in France. Chilled out I remember drinking too much alcohol, its purpose an attempt to forget the hurt that adopted us as orphans of normality, and fairness.

Sat 25th Feb 06: Went to Knightsbridge and visited Harrods together with John Lewis today but in all of this time uppermost in my thoughts, just how in god's name did we end up here, and what can we do?

Simple I thought, answer to the first question in our case, no safeguards within our NHS Blood Transfusion Service (at the time of Mark's transfusion no safeguards were in place for blood filtration) it was not until 1998, one year later that an attempt at filtration was tried. Despite the fact that during the BSE crisis Maternal prodigy (calves were being infected with CJD) even though they were taken away immediately after their birth circa 1992. It was of course a disease that was being passed on by bloods a vertical transmission, the government had known of the possible risks associated with TSE blood borne infection and its risks to humans since 1996 and before when the first recorded death to vCJD was announced, but they waited and waited watching the ball spin around their Roulette Wheel, gambling on it not landing on red ,but in 2003 it did exactly that, the first (recorded death to vCJD through a blood transfusion) Mr Kenny, but there may have been others before this, hidden from exposure, they perhaps trying to stall the inevitability of the eventual undeniable fact that BSE had crossed the human species barrier and into their precious now contaminated Blood Service!

We watched another show in London's Starry West End trying to lose ourselves in what seemed an ocean of pain, then limping to our senses made our way back to the realization of another night in a strange bed before that cold light of dawn that followed gave us a further hotel menu for breakfast.

Victoria Railway Station at lunchtime for me that day in Feb 2006 and its associated journey back to Brighton was not something I truly relished, taking a ride back to the everyday hell of losing my son, but what could I do?

Chapter Eight

Writing a Book

Then it came to me, that eureka moment; I would try and let as many people know as possible, we would form a type of militia, a revolutionary army and storm Westminster trying to inject a little common sense into a decision making party that had lost their way. Already some daily papers were aware of our family's monumental problem of being dealt the worst possible cards in the game of life, our dear son's life span now simply a matter of weeks away, his dementia accelerating like a time warp, into a space a place only Mark could go.

Instead I decided perhaps I would try and write a book (the easier option or so I thought)

Mon 27th Feb 2006: Workman arrived at our mews house in order to convert the bathroom into a wet room for our need to accommodate Mark's requirements for showering etc, also removing a stud wall between our two bedrooms on the second floor again making for a considerably larger space to accommodate his bed and a chance to place Mark's personal items around him, those we had collected from Ipswich.

Obviously we had to move out on a temporary basis and elected to stay at a hotel in Brighton with Mark.

Tues 28th Feb 2006: Came and went with settling in to our new accommodation, and all the problems that went with this phase of our difficult journey.

However I am blessed with a wife who is a super organiser, and for the most part took a fair bit of stress out of a dreadful situation.

Thurs 1st March 2006: Mark's counsellor comes down from London, and one of our son's friends visited.

Took my son wrapped up warmly against a cold Brighton blast and pushed him in his NHS wheelchair along the Brighton seafront being greeted only by a galaxy of Brighton seagulls forever eager to pluck a morsel from a non attentive participant's grasp, we got a cup of tea, I remembered also noticing now almost daily by how much more limited Mark's conversational ability was becoming.

Back at the hotel in the warm, Mark expressed a wish to use the internet so utilising the hotels Wi-Fi he spent some while e-mailing and I was very surprised how well he coped with this procedure.

Early evening saw me in the lounge of the hotel, my son resting and Eve chatting on her mobile stayed with our son watching all these individuals booking in and out of reception. It gave me some space and a little time to reflect on the history of how both Eve and I had arrived in 2006 at the foot of what seemed an unassailable and deeply challenging period of time.

I had first met Eve at a Xmas party way back in 1967 where we both worked for the same company at that time, a television rental business based in Hove near Brighton.

Eve in the office, and me servicing the televisions both in the field and sometimes within the workshops that lay within a Mews in Hove, I am not sure what magic spell she cast on me that day, when I first saw this curly brown headed figure in a black figure hugging dress, can't put a finger on the way my then comfortable and unchallenged existence screeched to a halt at one of life's crossroads, up until I had first met Eve I was that laid back bachelor personified.

I was that guy who hung around with my mates in the evenings, invariably in a pub somewhere, and shared a common experience in the smell of spilt beer and crackling crisp packets, of the vibrant renderings of the Rolling Stones or indeed any of the Top Ten tunes in what seemed then an endless supply of fervent sixties vocal energy that could be supplied at the touch of a juke box button.

There is a saying that everyone experiences a moment in their time on this earth that perhaps they need to grasp with both hands. A bit like the game of Monopoly when you can pass jail and collect £200 perhaps it's an intuitive instinct that's genetically a part of our brains software, but whatever it was on that late afternoon in December 1967 I felt its pull and was magnetically attracted to this girl dressed in black with a lovely smile and extraordinary organisational skills, that soft beckoning hauntingly, almost off limits female, I just needed more of the same, but did not altogether realize at the time just what I was getting into.

Eve is still blessed with the same skills 44 years later, and her personality totally opposite to mine, I have always worn my heart on my sleeve, and Eve will internalize most problems creating a calmer external influence as part of her personality.

Strangely we both got married twice, but to each other, the first occasion a civil ceremony in March 1969 in Hove's Registry Office, and then waited until January 1970, and a religious marriage in the city of London in Bevis Mark's synagogue EC3 the oldest Spanish and Portuguese synagogue in England circa 1701.

So these two celebrations marking the start of our married life together, in truth one I suppose much like a lot of other peoples, I know we both worked hard at, I remaining in the same trade as a TV engineer until I reached the age of 50 and Eve continued to work in between the births of our 3 children mainly in office work.

At 50 I had a career change when I had the opportunity to work within a school for deaf children servicing a requirement for their needs to maintain and improve an audible link to both the teaching staff and into the outside world, this school for the most part was a boarding school and set in a pleasant landscape east of Brighton centre. It was at this school that I was first advised in 2004 that Mark may be at risk of a tainted blood transfusion.

Thurs 2nd March 2006: Saw our now endlessly hurting bodies wake up to Brighton sunshine, and remember looking down from our hotel's window that overlooked the famous Brighton Pier watching the blue/grey waves invite their Ariel companions the herring gulls to rest awhile and digest whatever spoils they had managed to retrieve from the vast choice of plastic dustbin bags that were available in the many streets within this city.

Today we were driving to London by taxi to firstly visit The National Prion Clinic with our son and arrived at approx 4.30 that afternoon. Our appointment scheduled for the next day.

Mark having difficulty now with his mobile phone, his memory impairment increasing almost daily, it was a very difficult and testing time, just to think that in the past our son's immense skill levels in IT were second to none!

We stayed in the same hotel as we had done before adjacent to Queen Square; I noted the facilities for wheelchairs were less than perfect.

Fri 3rd March 2006: It was snowing that day as we made the short journey from hotel to the entrance of the hospital armed with nothing more than a sense of fear of the unknown.

Met Mark's girlfriend at the hospital, our youngest daughter was also at the meeting, together with a good family friend of ours Margaret Wood who was and still remains a very caring lady.

Various issues were discussed at the meeting which began at 10.30 that morning, any distant hopes regarding our son's future were soon kicked into touch. Mark in his wheelchair was now a mere spectator of life as we know it, every day now passing him by on the touch line of what had once been a competitive and successful career, his facial appearance increasingly betraying his illness.

We were all shown around the research and development space within this hospital, a unit dedicated to the cohort study of this prion disease, led by Prof John Collinge.

I remember Prof Collinge asking our son on that day, an IT question relating to a problem that their team had met with in their research of this disease, and Mark from his wheelchair, being both surprised and then thoughtful of this question, slowly answered him. I was so proud of Mark's reply at this late stage of his regression and reversely so tearful and saddened by his status of a disabled astronaut about to be launched into a void from where no traveller returns and can you even imagine how it feels to be a parent in this crisis.

What I needed right then was a stiff drink, my spaceship into oblivion, but then I looked around and saw that nobody else wanted to follow me they were all stronger and yes I was ashamed of my own obvious weakness, the unashamedly open path I followed towards alcoholism, for me a need to escape the reality of what I knew by then to mean I was about to witness the death of my only beautiful son.

We eventually departed Queen Square in favour of Heathrow Airport. A taxi organised by the hospital drove Mark and myself, together with Eve and her friend Margaret towards an airport hotel and another holiday destination for our dear son.

After a fairly comfortable but nevertheless noisy journey we arrived at the wrong hotel. Ah yes there are two Sheraton Hotels within a short distance of Heathrow and our driver managed to deliver all four of us complete with wheelchair to the wrong one. Having arrived at the incorrect reception desk at the wrong hotel, we were rerouted to the correct destination via another taxi and before collecting our thoughts found ourselves ensconced within rather plush surroundings at our eventual correct destination. Another round of alcohol.

Of thoughts that came in the night, of hopes that were continually smashed into oblivion, nightmares that remain and plenty more besides, hey, well what do you expect a happy ending?

Breakfast was good the next morning, Mark appears ok. Another taxi, another day. Terminal 1 was this destination's mission and a group of very good friends about to share maybe a final celebration of our son's life, a chance to have that group hug but more than that to say goodbye in whatever language they chose.

Arrived Terminal 1, and our son met with his close friends, their flight was 11.15 to Palma, as Eve and I said another goodbye to Mark, we both knew this was likely to be the very last time he was going to be able to interact with any real clarity with his friends before a large neuronal invasion overshadowed completely normality as he had once known it.

Next stop was another airport, in name Gatwick, on arriving at the end of another taxi journey we booked ourselves into a Hilton Hotel had a meal and over dinner had a text from Mark with a question: What had been the make of his very first car? I struggled to remember and then replied. Had a beer and then reflected on the next day, we were flying to Malta and getting the ferry across to the island of Gozo, we couldn't be at home because of the workmen carrying out conversions etc. to the house, and so to bed.

Good flight to Malta and arriving finally at Ta-Tench Hotel on Gozo we collapsed by the pool side and studied the evening menu, looked at Mark's website and saw he was enjoying himself, could relax a little more now.

Another day on the island of Gozo and all of the time thinking of Mark, and trying not to visualize too far ahead, it is far too painful a process.

The days flew by as invariably they do when on holiday, and every day the shadows lengthened but they seemed darker than usual mirroring my innermost thoughts and taunting the inevitable acceptance of Mark's decline.

Sat 11th March 2006: Back home and busy tidying up after builders had completed both bedroom and wet room conversions, fitting shelves and replacement units to suit, kept me both busy and my mind off some of the hurt that was always lurking.

I found myself shouting at Eve and she said, "Why are you so angry?"

"Why," I said, "is because my son is dying!"

So much easier now that our son's bedroom was a decent size and could now accommodate most of his personal items; computer, hi-fi etc.

The wet room was another triumph and was a great blessing in an aid to meet Mark's increasing needs. Well done Margaret Leitch for both the drive and dedication you provided in our time of need.

Sun 12th March: Our eldest daughter's birthday today, and Mark returns from his Spanish holiday. It was lovely to see him again but even in the short time he had been away the poor kid had regressed a tad more.

Sunday 12th March: Arranged for Mark to visit Martlets Hospice Tues next.

Today Monday 13th: Eve had been busy organising again, and together with care co-ordinators arranged as much as was possible towards maximizing at this late stage all the requirements for our son's needs.

Day nurses had an input in our lives together with probably at this stage of Mark's illness an ever increasing requirement for night nursing.

Daily Hallifax Care provided practical care and support to our family.

Providing an invaluable service for our son's declining health, something which freed time up for us to organise and develop other special needs in this crisis.

Tues 14th March 2006: Our wedding anniversary and I remember with a deal of regret forgetting this moment in time, neither Eve or I mentioned it.

Eve in London for some much earned therapy, leaving Mark and myself to explore the day as it unfolded.

Another new symptom arrives on Mark's battlefield, his inability to swallow is now a big concern, to combat this problem we need to thicken Mark's drinks.

Eve is the main informal carer for our son, Mark has experienced several falls and we are concerned about the night time when we are downstairs.

We had recently heard a loud noise from upstairs at night, only to find Mark on the floor, we needed to constantly monitor Mark when he was alone at night in his bedroom, and it was to this end I finally installed an infrared camera one end of his room in order to monitor his safety, later on this proved an invaluable aid for the night nurse.

Eve always busy supervising his meals and administering Mark's medication, we are also discovering that Mark is spending more time asleep now and needs motivation.

We are currently awaiting a motability car as we have to rely either on ambulances or specially adapted vehicles to transport Mark anywhere. Currently Mark attends the Martlets Day Centre on a Tuesday but this was to increase as time went on.

Wed 15th March: Mark has a nasty cough, called GP out and Mark is now on antibiotics. Another person arrives into Mark's life this time a speech therapist, as this disease progresses our son is starting to have swallowing problems and his speech is noticeably becoming slurred, poor bastard as if he hasn't gone through enough!

Today another meeting in Brighton to further discuss our son's case and his needs.

Speech therapist spends time with Mark today.

And so the days go by, Mark's friends come and go, and the reason some are nameless and not included in this book is at their specific request.

A new bed support for Mark arrives, his support team very active in all directions.

Sat 18th March 06: Haven't written for a few days I am finding it difficult trying to do justice to this story, Mark's regression inevitable it's not an easy path for any of us, Mark's girlfriend came down from Ipswich and stayed overnight, Mark of course enjoyed that, she is a very upbeat young woman.

A new workman on site at our house in the form of a representative from Stannah stair lifts who were measuring our property in order that our son could traverse the two floors to his bedroom in a more sane and less stressful way.

Another symptom develops in that Mark now occasionally has rapid hand movements I think when he feels stressed and it's an increasing problem.

Trying to get out on my bike a little now, it's a great stress buster and in 20 minutes from our village mews you could find yourself on the South Downs way with picture postcard views and a chance to get away briefly from the nightmare our poor son, and family were going through. I don't know personally how else I could have coped, without my trusty Dave Yates road bike, pushing my mentally stressed body mile after mile on my red racer, temporarily detaching my mind from the hopelessness of our son's unrelenting and impending entrance to the black hole that unthinking policy makers had designed for him. Mark also when he had been well was a keen cyclist, a much stronger one than me I add, on his Harry Hall blue painted road bike, regularly putting in a lot of miles and enjoying his escape, his chance to burn off some free radicals, and to taste the triumph of climbing that big hill, and to feel your often spent body recover moments later, and a chance to shake some lactic acid from your tired legs, speeding towards home, only to do it all again the next day, it was until recently a best kept secret amongst enthusiasts and club riders, but thankfully I suppose more people are enjoying the amazing benefits of cycling now and long may it continue.

Mon 20th March 06: Found Eve and I at the International Conference on CJD held in London at BMA house in upper Woburn Place, we had travelled up the previous day as it was to be an early start on Monday and stayed at a Hilton Hotel adjacent to the conference hall.

I remember tabling a question for the panel that day, finding it all a bit tame wanting to, preferring to, direct my questions to the government and its associated health ministers.

My question aimed at the National Blood Service and its associated Consultant Specialist, a Dr Patricia Hewitt.

The question was simple: "Could she tell me what progress had been made since 1998 and the first introduction of an attempt at Prion filtration in the form of Leucoreduction? Since two definite cases of prion infection via blood transfusions had resulted one in death and the other by detection at autopsy (this last case dying of another cause). Mark of course was to be the next victim. If I can remember Leucoreduction only offered something like a 42% chance of working by the (quote) removal of white cells from blood, the other step that had been put into place was stopping the use of fractioned blood in Plasma products and obtaining supplies of fresh frozen Plasma (for children only) from non UK sources. More importantly there is a necessity to remove the remaining non-cell associated infectivity.

Excluding donors who could be at increased risk of vCJD, i.e. those who have themselves received blood transfusions (unquote).

I got the distinct understanding that it was a lack of funding, but what price is a life I asked myself.

The problem with this is unless the Blood Service within the UK can guarantee to have traceability of every tainted recipient or donor of bloods then it simply is gambling with peoples' lives. And what is more there is evidence that this case scenario has happened in the past!

Ever since the death of my son to vCJD via a tainted blood transfusion in 2006 I have been pushing the government for an effective blood filtration system to be introduced within the UK, in the year 2009 there were two such devices available, the P-CAPT prion capture filter by MacoPharma being one such device with an efficacy of 99.9% reduction of exogenous brain spike infectivity in red blood cell concentrates. And 90% reduction of endogenous whole blood infectivity globally, over 90 million blood units are collected annually and this is a solution, but remains one that is not adopted by our Tory Government.

Chapter Nine

Failings within Governmental Health

Despite more than one visit to no 10 Downing St, and the handing in of letters regarding the need for greater safeguards within our UK Blood Transfusion Service, and subsequent meetings both in Westminster and with my local MP any adoption of such a very fundamental and vital service remains to date Nov 2013 unadopted and one to which only lip service has been paid.

Below is a list of some of the large number of committed health professionals needed in the last few months of my sons life.

GP's (excluding those in Ipswich)
Neurologist (ditto)
District Nurses
Sitting Services
Speech and Language therapist
Occupational Therapist
Physiotherapist
Psychologist
Palliative Care Specialist
Palliative care Nurse
Psychiatrist
Complementary Therapist
Dentist
Counselling

The majority of vCJD patients require 24 hour nursing.

None of the above could hope to save Mark, however in our darkest hours they all played a very significant part in guiding our family in a very sympathetic and caring fashion.

When you consider that in spite of the government's own Advisory Service on Blood Tissue and Organs SABTO recommending the aforementioned filtration system nothing has moved forward (except the withdrawal of this Advisory Committees Funding) (good isn't it.)

At this conference I had the chance to speak with other vCJD affected families and learnt at first hand of their particular circumstances and involvement, I could of course easily identify with their often courageous battles.

My mobile rang during the lunch break, a message from Stannah stair lifts advising me that the lift that they were attempting to fit that day in our house in Brighton and that was so necessary to us, simply did not fit it was mis-measured and therefore could not be fitted, I was very upset at the thought of poor Mark having to struggle up two flights of stairs any longer and immediately handed the problem onto the Claymore wielding lassie from Scotland Mrs Margaret Leitch the National CJD Surveillance's Care Co-ordinator, she had always been a tower of strength to our family and I speak as I find.

Needless to say on our return that day from our meeting in London Margaret had managed to persuade the stair lift Co to make a temporary fitting and to return at a later date to refit another, job done and a great relief especially for dear Mark who must have thought it a godsend. To ascend and descend those two flights at the touch of a button.

One of the many people I had met that day at the conference was Mr Peter Mills whose lovely daughter Holly had contracted vCJD.

Peter had adopted a drug that is called Pentosan Polysulphate or (PPS), it is derived from Beechwood and has anti inflammatory properties.

Some experimental results can be summarised as indicating that PPS has effects on prion protein, replication and associated cell toxicity.

PPS unfortunately does not cross the blood-brain barrier after oral administration and so intraventricular administration is needed to deliver the drug to the brain.

A brave decision to make in my humble opinion since there were risks involved with surgery however clearly to date Mr Peter Mills made the correct decision in that as a direct result of this procedure his lovely daughter Holly went on to live for a considerable amount of time (unfortunately since writing this chapter Holly Mills has passed away).

To this day I am not sure whether I should have taken this option as well, however it was not an option that was available under Professor Collinge, he could only offer the drug Quinacrine in a clinical trial, since Pentosan was only offered under a special license and through a court hearing and frowned upon by government. I simply didn't want to put my son through any more trauma. Conversely if in the year 2000 when it had first became known that Mark may be at risk of vCJD because one of his blood donors died of vCJD, yes of course we would have used the drug PPS, but as I have already mentioned the DOH said nothing to warn us of our son's at risk assessment, hoping perhaps it would never happen, another roulette wheel, gambling with other peoples' lives had been I suggest a part of their agenda for so long they failed to see the wood for the trees.[5]

It is important to realise that the current treatment of humans with CJD is a treatment being given (after) the actual onset of clinical disease. If a treatment is efficacious in progressive neurological disease, then it is very reasonable to believe that the sooner it is given, the better the positive results.

Therefore it is very important that patients seeking treatment with PPS be given it as early as possible.

In simple terms I think it true to say that had Mark taken this drug orally in the year 2000 instead of having to wait until 2006 and beyond and before a clinical invasion of his central nervous system i.e. before it had crossed his blood brain

---

[5] In some instances, animals in experimental infection appear to be completely protected from the development of disease Dr RSG Knight on potential treatments for CJD. 2005.

barrier, there was a chance he would have survived. So there we have it in a Nutshell.

1. Our son transfused with a tainted blood product in 1997.
2. A failure by the DOH to advise our son that he may be at risk of vCJD in 2000 when it first became known that he may be at risk.
3. A complete failure by his designated neurologist to take a local clinical lead in assessing and providing advice for the person at risk other than advise Mark there was 1 in a million chance of him being infected in Jan 2004.
4. A failure on the part of his GP to link his recorded symptoms with his eventual warning that he may be at risk of vCJD in Jan 2004.
5. A complete failure by all those that were involved in decision making regarding our son's known at risk status from April 2000 through to 2006.
6. Below a list of culpable bodies that sadly failed Mark.
7. The Department of Health to decide whether any recipient of a tainted blood transfusion should be told or not)! their object (the PAR may commit suicide) I think not.
8. Mark's designated neurologist in Ipswich who failed to pick up on or follow up on Mark's early signs of vCJD despite DOH warning.
9. Mark's GP in Ipswich who failed to recognise our son's classic vCJD symptoms until Dec 05 despite his symptoms and her knowledge of his at risk status in Jan 2004 and the publications on early symptoms of vCJD that had been available since 2001 and before.
10. As a result of my son's Coroner's Inquest the coroner was sufficiently moved to report his findings to the dept of health, as a result of this an 18 page report was published by members of the vCJD Clinical Governance Advisory Group and chaired by Sir William Stewart.

11. Amongst its recommendations. The condition of the person at risk should be reviewed by the GP and designated neurologist if symptoms of concern develop (Within Mark's medical notes lots of history of early symptoms of vCJD) that went undetected as vCJD.

Monday 20th March 06: Whilst Eve and I were in London Mark went to his friends gated Mews property in the Marina at Brighton, he visited the local supermarket whilst there and for Mother's Day bought Eve a card, in spite of all his insurmountable problems his true character of always thinking of other people shone through.

Tues 21st March 06: Mark's double bed installed to include a back riser, representative from Stannah Lifts returns and carefully re-measures stair lift.
More of Mark's friends visit and a lot of these visitors lived a fair way out of Brighton. And so our son's life continued but for how long no one could be sure.

Wed 22nd March: Today two visitors from London's Prion Clinic arrived monitoring our son's failing condition, came down from London.

Thurs 23rd March 06: Mark visited two dear friends they had dinner followed I understand by chocolate cake.
Our son continues despite all the crap that he has to confront every day.

Fri 24th March 06: Mark's girlfriend visits with her parents from Ipswich, I remember she tickled his feet whilst he went up the stairs in his chairlift and made Mark laugh, he was always very happy when his girlfriend was around.

Sat 25th March 06: Mark's two sisters gave our son a head and foot massage, and another old friend Sam visited. Lots of visitors today.

Sun 26th March 06: Mother's Day found our family lunching in the county town of Lewes, at The White Hart Hotel we had pre booked and there was adequate room for Mark's wheelchair.

Mark had a good day, looked relaxed, it was a perfect day. I am hoping shortly to receive a Motobility Vehicle it's a little testing for Mark and his wheelchair to squeeze into my little Polo.

Mon 27th March 06: Mark's counsellor comes down from London at midday, and wrote this to Mark after they had returned from a trip into Brighton. 'Thank you for a lovely afternoon, we will have to go to Wan a Kik a Moo Kow again,' (this a Café in the North Laines in Brighton) 'for ice-cream, and play more table football'. She was a valuable contributor in counselling Mark when it mattered most.

Chapter Ten

Celebrating Mark's Life

Tues 28th March 06: Mark's 32nd birthday and a surprise party for Mark at the Metropole Hotel on Brighton's seafront.

A very happy and emotional day for all concerned, knowing this was likely to be the very last birthday he would ever get to celebrate was a strong reminder of just where our son was in life's cycle of sometimes tragic proportion.

Lots of dear friends, lots of chocolate, which Mark of course loved, balloons, laughter, our eldest daughter had come up from Devon with her children.

I can remember videoing a part of that celebration that day and together with lots of other footage captured at different times of his so short a life, my brother in law Van editing and releasing a DVD of Mark's life from two to thirty two.

Wed 29th March 06: One of Mark's good friends here at our mews house sorting out Mark's computer etc. She is over from Australia, and retrieving photographs from files on his PC. As you may remember our son had been a very keen and competent photographer from an early age and had stored a lot of these images on his computer's hard drive.

The plan was to give our Mark a photographic exhibition at Proud St Galleries in London. And combine that with a stay at the Savoy Hotel which was a stone's throw away from the planned exhibition. And along with other friends she was instrumental in setting up the exhibition, I know it was organised beautifully and was a resounding success.

But more of that later. Mark and his girlfriend return from a night at the Hilton Hotel after breakfast in bed and a relaxing shower.

Eve booked the Savoy Hotel for family and friends together with a stretch limo to take us up in style.

Thurs 30th March 06: "Savoy Hotel please," I instructed the stretch limo driver in my most casual voice, I don't think the driver was too happy since he had tried for some while to manoeuvre his newly valeted leather seated London bound missile into our cramped mews entrance deciding after what seemed an eternity to park in the narrow road outside of the mews was the only option, and his face a picture when he also realised that Mark's wheelchair was to be his front seat passenger. We all eventually got seated and when our chauffeur's face had turned back from crimson to a more natural pinkish colour I asked him after a short way up the A23, "Could I open a bottle of champagne?" I took the grunt to mean a yes, and as I was quite adept at this sort of thing, well on my way to becoming a connoisseur of wine by this stage (Eve called me a piss artist) which in truth was a nearer description of where I had got to, proceeded to pour our Mark a glass.

It was Mark's mum who instantly said, "He can't drink that he is on tablets."

At which Mark replied, "Fuck the Tablets!" and in an embarrassingly short time had consumed his glass of iced Moet Chan don. I of course followed instantly, relaxing into the white leather seats happily gazing through tinted windows one eye on the other unopened champagne bottles and one on watching Mark close his eyes and going wherever his irreparable increasingly[6] floral plaqued brain was taking him.

Arrived very grandly at the Savoy Hotel, our driver having to reverse his car passengers who included my wife, yours truly, our eldest daughter, her children, Mark of course and his wheelchair plus luggage up to the eagerly awaiting door men.

We were ushered into some of the most luxurious surroundings through oak glazed brass adorned and fit for a prince doors, our luggage remaining the sole responsibility of

---

[6] Floral plaques in Brain Autopsy are recognisable indications of vCJD.

the Savoy staff resplendent in their Savoy livery, we were soon shown our respective rooms sampling what most millionaires would count as just another day at the office.

Thursday afternoon in the Savoy was sumptuous and reassuringly grand enough for me to relax a little and lower my guard a tad.

With Mark's girlfriend joining us at the Savoy our son was now as relaxed and happy as he could ever be in his now fucked up world.

And so on Thursday 30th March 06 the desperately hurting Buckland family sought shelter in one of London's famous hotels, seeking refuge from a hurt that dominated every thought, every crevice of my spatial awareness, my only temporary escape another drink or two, like a temporary filling in an aching tooth where I knew the pain perhaps would only stop when that part of my life was removed completely. I was to find that analogy false, despite all of the heartache knowing we would shortly lose such an important part of our lives, it was and remains more of a loss since we closed his coffin now just an empty void, an untouchable precious star.

I marvelled at the opulence, the fancy frills, the extra deep carpet, must have walked the entire length and breadth of its ever curvy twisting seemingly endless corridors, got drunk on passing ladies Chanel no5 and other deeply sensual experiences that seemed to have filled this hotel's stairways like shadows from its past, went and had a look at the rather suave cocktail bar but in truth was put off by its pricey bar menu, but I knew of another bar, in the form of my suitcase and returned there to open a bottle of chateau de unwins, and sipping this wine which tasted remarkably decent from the bathroom glass after I had removed the toothbrushes of its previous occupants, reflected on the day and fell asleep Savoy style.

Friday 31st March 06: Woke to a marble shower room, a wife who was showered, dressed and was impatient for me to join her for breakfast.

A lot to do today and we went over the many tasks that were planned over a Savoy silver service breakfast.

Eldest daughter had an appointment at the MRC Prion Clinic, an opportunity she readily took since she rarely was able to visit London from her home city of Exeter.

That appointment was pencilled in for 11.30 that morning.

Busy, bustling, foyer, everyone jostling for prime position at the reception desk, competent staff with welcoming smiles, where Louis Vuitton luggage and Savile Row suits are commonplace and the expectancy of a sanctuary par-excellence is assured, I cried silent tears when I saw my Mark in his NHS wheelchair on a tour of the hotel's many rooms, you see in spite of where he was in life he could still smile that smile that was 'a bute' as our Australian cousins might say.

Daughter left with her husband for Queen Square and the Neurological Hospital to get up to speed with her brother's condition.

Eve and I took the boys out to Hamleys Toy Shop and I remember I treated them each to a toy of their choice, and a third for our Mark knowing his passion for robotics, we purchased him a remotely controlled robot; it turned out to be a fascinating distraction for him. It remains to this day stored lovingly in my bedroom wardrobe, a nostalgic link to an irreplaceable person whose long and winding road lay mined, not by the Alkiada but Governmental incompetence.

On our return to the hotel we met up with those friends of Mark's who had been so diligent in organising the main reason we were in London this weekend. Mark's photographic exhibition that was to be held at the Proud Galleries in John Adam Street WC2, a short walk from our chosen hotel.

One of Mark's good friends as I had mentioned previously had been mainly instrumental in organising which photographs that were held on Mark's PC were to be processed in order that they may be hung in this exhibitions gallery, and after some deliberation with Mark and other friends, chose a number of diverse images that highlighted an enduring ability to capture a simple purity in an increasingly complex world.

Mark's aim was to attract the viewers' attention whilst allowing them enough space to reflect upon this image.

The exhibition was called LIGHT and was his first and tragically last time to shine as a very competent photo artist.

There was to be two viewings, the first a ticket only affair today in the evening, times 7 till 9pm, and tomorrow Saturday 10am until 4pm opened to the public.

It took a lot of organising by a number of enthusiastic and dedicated friends from all parts of the country who displayed a collective enthusiasm to celebrate his life despite what little time our son now had ahead of him.

Whilst the day was an extremely busy one we as a family found time to organise a high tea within the Savoy and family and friends were asked to join us in the afternoon. I remember capturing that scene on my video camera and it was reproduced latterly on a final DVD edited by Van my brother in law as a tribute to our son's all too brief a time on planet earth.

So there we have it, a gathering of friends and family and a new edition in the form of a monochrome walking talking robot who strutted his stuff on thick Savoy carpet and amused Mark just as we hoped it would.

The exhibition was a triumph and our son although insidiously regressing was really surprisingly focused as he was pushed around the exhibition in a form of transport that was so necessary to life as he knew it now, I so desperately wanted to understand what Mark may be thinking, of how he thought others may perceive him or maybe such thoughts were hidden from his brain's menu, now much modified by a man made misformed protein.

The exhibition was well attended with visitors coming great distances and the images well received, the wine was sipped, orders for copies of the prints were taken, I for one was proud and slightly humbled by the refreshing enthusiasm of everyone who took part and attended the occasion of a culmination of Mark's enthusiasm for photography and I suppose a final curtain bow to a hobby that he had taken to his heart from an early age, it was slightly melancholy to see him in the winter of his short life clinging on to his camera, guarding it as if his life depended on it, with always that certain smile that most times left my eyes moist.

Always trying to find a more pleasurable direction in the latter part of Mark's life was sometimes challenging but fine tuning Mark's resonant happy curve to a peak could easily be accomplished whenever his girlfriend was in close attendance.

Friday night 10pm arrived and as we exited Proud Galleries it was time to reflect on a very good evening at John Adam St in London's WC2 and look forward to more of the same the next day, but we had another surprise for Mark, another chance to see him enjoy himself before the Grim Reaper has to visit him and snatch a part of us and our life away forever.

Saturday 1st April 06: Awoke fairly early but not nearly early enough for Eve, she in her wisdom had slipped away to an early breakfast, and a seat in the restaurant that overlooked the Thames, always an early bird that catches the worm except her worm had been substituted for a gorgeous plate of fresh fruit. I chose as I invariably do in a decent restaurant poached haddock and if I could have got away with it a flute of fine champagne, instead I settled for a coffee and extra toast. I was joined by my eldest daughter accompanied by the only slightly muted tones of my grandchildren looking for anything that was disgustingly sweet and chocolate enhanced, their faces betraying the pleasure they found in a Savoy breakfast that was guaranteed to please.

Saturday continued where Friday had left off, with the continuation of Mark's Photographic Exhibition only now the doors were open to the public and we were all pleasantly surprised at the amount of bodies that passed through the doors and showed a genuine interest in our son's portfolio.

An enthusiastic audience made it all worthwhile, Van was videoing the event and some of the clips put to good use on an edit finishing as a treasured memory of our son's time.

If the morning was a rewarding and significantly important one then the afternoon needed to be different and fun.

So we collected Mark and his wheelchair together with our family and several friends and made our way to the London Eye, Eve had pre-booked a pod and very slowly with a lot of mirth we all completed a revolution.

For just one moment as we reached the highest part of the cycle I could clearly see Westminster and cursed those ministers who had shortened my son's life and that of many others with the amplification of BSE and it's crossover to vCJD.

Mark I was never so sure had really enjoyed his revolution, his time with friends, whose only goal was to make the most of what Mark had left a pleasurable experience, to not allow him to go raging into that night.

To be honest I am still hostile to the stupidity of the conservative regime and it's many broken promises, another good example occurred today as I write these pages, another postponement of the second hearing of the blood contaminated bill, the question on everyone's lips will this most important issue ever be addressed in Parliament with any conviction? I doubt it!

Saturday evening arrived after we had said our goodbyes to all those people who had made Mark's weekend special, and ate some pizza. I remember giving our son's girlfriend a break and sat with Mark in his hotel room. Mark was asleep, a prominent symptom of his illness, I remember thinking where do we go from here, what do I do now, when of course all of the time we were all just mere spectators of the passing of a very special person, nothing to do but rage at the unfairness of it all, and through the mist of pain try to imagine a life without him.

My mind wandering trying to hang on to past memories of my son and to relive those special times, it was my crack cocaine, my way of coping ,with a hurt that was so unbearable only alcohol could put me somewhere else.

Mark's girlfriend returns, and I immediately return to the bar of my choice in the form of a red suitcase that still contained a little chateau de unwins in my hotel room.

After saying goodnight to family and friends and watching the world go by sitting in the foyer of the Savoy, I took the lift and allowed nature to take over and a chance for a while to forget everything.

Sunday 2nd April 06: My birthday and to kick start it a silver service breakfast overlooking the Thames, I thrived on distractions, had made it down early that morning, I remember Mark having breakfast in his room together with his girlfriend, and gradually the table I had chosen filling up with my family and friends, this beautifully white laundered tablecloth not only sharing it's space with silverware, and best bone china, sat only slightly embarrassed by my gifts and birthday cards adorning it, a tribute to me reaching the grand old age of 62.

We sat and discussed the day ahead which I suppose for me was always going to be a bit of an anti-climax, in truth a hard three days to follow.

Having said our goodbyes and paying the bill, we were swept up again in our white stretch limo, with one extra passenger now; our youngest daughter. With happy memories of three days in London, a family mentally wounded and desperate to hold on to their Mark for as long as it was humanly possible made its way back to our village mews in Brighton.

Preparing for whatever lay ahead was difficult and always hoping for as much time as was possible with Mark was in my prayers constantly.

Monday 3rd April 06: Kat one of Mark's closest friends visits with some sad news, she has to return to Aussie, we will all miss her terribly as she is a really good friend to Mark.

Youngest daughter visits and they had dinner together.

Chapter Eleven

A Time for Peace

Tues 4th April 06: A visit to Martlets Hospice for Mark, and some time spent with his speech therapist again, a friend from London in the afternoon, and so this drama continued with care staff coming and going, friends doing the same all of us not knowing for just how much longer Mark could hang on.

Friday 7th: A day we had all been waiting for, the arrival of our son's mobility van, I was instructed in how to utilise all of its many functions by the delivery driver, then after signing the necessary papers, we were given a parking spot within our small mews by a very friendly neighbour who gave up his spot so that we could park this reasonably large Mercedes mobility van without a problem.

A huge plus for Mark no longer confined to squeezing often awkwardly into a normal vehicle but now able to remain when mobile in his wheelchair and after producing a list of designated drivers Mark had the luxury of a choice of various friends who were able then to be more flexible with whatever journeys Mark needed to take. I remember then taking Mark with a good friend of his university days for a trip up to a famous beauty spot which lay only a short distance from our home in Preston village, we arrived at a spot called Ditchling Beacon a high vantage point to which there is an awe-inspiring view of the many villages of Sussex and beyond. It was a pleasant sunny day, we struggled to make any real progress along the ruts of the Southdown way, his NHS red painted wheelchair groaning a path westerly through a blaze of meadow flowers finally halting at what seemed a good vantage point for a view. I then asked my son whether he could detail the view we were gazing on, and was gobsmacked when he recalled the names of the villages below us, we looked upon a rook filled Stanmer woods except now that wood perhaps seemed to me was more like Great Birnham wood and the hill we stood on was no longer Ditchling Beacon but Dunsimane hill although no witches could be seen, the skylarks remained singing their bewitching song above us. I remember thinking I love you Mark, the fragility of his situation forever uppermost in my mind.

Day by day Mark was slowly getting more distant but everyone connected with Mark remained totally supportive and interacted in a very caring manner.

Mark now thinks if asked his age that he is 22 not 32, a sure sign of increasing damage to his frontal lobe!

Our son's legs are noticeably and steadily getting weaker, but Mark I am sure also realizes the extent of his failing health and puts on a resigned front especially to his close friends.

The Stannah stair lift company returns and reinstall the lift so now it's a perfect fit, so a big thanks to them.

Mark is able to be pushed in his wheelchair in a large park almost opposite our mews house; the park is called Preston Park and is situated alongside the A23 as you enter Brighton.

Monday 10th April 06: Youngest daughter went to Martlets Hospice today with Mark and he drank a glass of Bucks Fizz. I'm not sure where he got that from, he then played a game of cards winning because apparently he was cheating and when the ward sister went out of the room he asked his sister to join him in cheating.

Very funny really, he then told his sister his age which was always 10 years younger and when his sister reminded Mark of his real age his reply he said, "Oh fuck you are right," much to the consternation of the elderly ladies surrounding him.

This another sad reminder of how a young man was left with dementia as perhaps a person in their late eighties or nineties may have been, it was heartbreaking but we had no choice other than to be witnesses to this fatal disease and simply be spectators of his impending demise, the contents of the poisoned cauldron had decided he had lived long enough.

Tues 11th April: A very close friend visits and has dinner, she interacts brilliantly with our son and was a former flat mate of Mark's when they were both at Manchester University.

And so a constant stream of people coming and going and all of the time I am sure it cheered Mark up enormously to see people caring.

April was an extraordinarily busy month for everyone involved with our son's care, everything had now been put into place to maximise whatever time was left to Mark on this earth, except no one could halt the invasive and relentless march of variant CJD, and its associated mis-folded prions.

The visitations to Martlets Hospice were now getting more frequent week by week, it was now thought by the local health authority to be where Mark would spend his final time and to get him accustomed to its surroundings was an important aspect of their dealing with our son's sometimes understandably confused sense of where he was, and at what stage of his rapidly declining health he would be admitted to this very important final resting place for the very sick, nestled as it is on the outskirts of Hove was just a matter of time.

Our daughters were now spending as much time together with my grandchildren and Mark as possible in sharing his exponentially declining decay curve heading rapidly towards its final ending.

April turned to May and continued to be crazily active, Mark now decidedly losing more of his central nervous functions and managed to try and enter an airing cupboard mistaking it for the toilet door.

It had been suggested in early May as a result I think of a meeting between some health professionals and Mark's close friends and further endorsed by Mark that perhaps Eve and I should take a short break and go away somewhere on holiday.

Martlets Hospice was getting to know our son more and more by now, although he seemed a lot easier when he was accompanied by a friend.

On Sat 13th May, Eve and I took a break to the Isle of Capri leaving our dear son was difficult but he seemed to be coping and was surrounded by an army of carers and friends, to make it easier and we thought safer he was to have respite care whilst Eve and I were away, in Martlets Hospice.

Monday 15th May: Mark accompanied by several friends left his mews retreat for Martlets Hospice where he was going just for a short stay, or so we all thought.

Eve and I were away at this junction but had been confident enough of his daily health and of the Martlets staff and his endless friends, of doctors that visited from London, to feel reassured of his temporary well being whilst we were absent.

From a diary that our youngest daughter kept during our absence he was surrounded with love and care but noticed on Tuesday 16th Mark had been sick in the night.

On the Wednesday speech therapist visited, several friends in attendance, in afternoon Dr's from London visited as well as Mark's social worker.

On the same day and over 1740 kilometres away in a hotel under a blue sky and relaxing alongside a sun drenched pool on the isle of Capri, Mark's parents were alerted by hotel reception to a telephone call from one of our son's friends.

My heart skipped a beat or two, at the same time alarm bells rang loudly, a dull narcotic sense of foreboding filled me with dread when it was explained to me that we needed to return as soon as possible because Mark was deteriorating fast.

I thanked this person and made immediate arrangements to get the next flight home which was to be later that day chucking all our clothes etc into relevant suitcases we arranged both a taxi to the island's small port and then by boat to the mainland and in all of this time hoping we would make it back in time, chastising ourselves for ever leaving him in the first place we spent the next few hours travelling and eventually boarding our flight back to the UK and our dear son Mark Adam Buckland.

It was Thursday 18th May early morning when we next saw Mark and I did detect a change in him although I was encouraged by his only slightly suppressed smile, his ward filled with family and friends, my eldest daughter and family were now in Brighton I do believe they had had a similar phone call in Exeter and had travelled up to be with Mark.

I am this moment looking at the list of people who visited Mark in the hospice from the 18th May and until the 23rd May.

Dozens of well-wishers; friends and family, advisors doctors, our local Rabbi.

His ward had a waiting list, constantly queuing, I think everyone sensing Mark's frailness and a need to perhaps say goodbye in their own way.

As Friday came and went my heart grew heavier, as a father I sensed an ending and I hated it and it got a lot worse, although everything in place for our son's care including massages for Mark as much upbeat joviality that could be expected it was all going on in down town Martlets.

Monday 22nd May: Lee an old friend sitting with Mark playing a repertoire of tunes on his guitar.

A phone call from Texas for Mark.

He was still hanging on, good boy Mark I thought but winced at what lay ahead.

And then Monday evening just family left in Mark's ward and I have repeated nightmares of this moment, I was the last to leave the ward, giving my dear son just a little more liquid in the form of a smoothie, he seemed thirsty. I kissed him goodbye and proceeded to walk to the entrance of the hospice as I trod the corridor and reached my eldest daughter who was waiting just outside I knew it was nearly all over for Mark. I broke down and sobbed on my daughter's shoulder at the darkness that was closing in for my beautiful son.

Tuesday 23rd May 06: Awoken by an early phone call from Martlets, "Please come quickly Mark is failing." We contacted our daughters immediately and sped towards the hospice, but we were too late, he had just breathed for the very last time.

Our precious son had left us at 7.10 that Tuesday morning. He had gone where there was no suffering, no longer in a space restricted by a brain wasting disease that slowly stripped the very essence of who Mark was and spat it out, our son god rest his soul couldn't go on any longer, he finally gave up his fight to an incurable disease that was a direct result of a tainted blood transfusion within the NHS. A legacy of the witches' cauldron.

When my eldest daughter arrived at the hospital she was visually upset and our whole perception of life was now challenged and distorted, life as we had previously known it could never be the same, he was our star, truly a man of worth.

We all had a short time alone with Mark as he lay on his hospice bed still warm to the touch; his presence in this world for those people lucky enough to have known him was now going to be just a treasured memory.

Arrangements have to be made when people pass away, everybody knows that, however if we ever thought that the worst was over we were totally wrong.

Our Rabbi was contacted, funeral arrangements made, in the Jewish religion it's traditional that the burial takes place within 48 hours of the death of a person. I believe this tradition goes back to Biblical times and beyond when because of the very hot climate in the Middle East it was necessary to bury the dead person as quickly as possible to avoid fast decomposition of remains.

Tuesday as you can imagine was a very stressful day in trying to organise all that was needed to be accomplished in the preparation of Mark's funeral.

But like just about every other obstacle that the Buckland family had to overcome in the preceding months this was never going to be any different.

A representative from the National Prion Cohort Clinic in Queen Square arrived with some papers to sign, Mark was to have an autopsy before burial could be considered!

Ok you say, fair enough, except these were the conditions we as a family had to agree to, now are you comfortable then listen carefully to these stipulations as laid out by Dr Wroe, yes the same neurologist who first spoke to our son in January 2004!

The autopsy that was to be carried out in Brighton was I believe a shared one between London and a local surgeon.

What was requested was the complete removal of Mark's brain (or what was left of it) I believe for research, fair enough you might say except in our religion that is not acceptable.

I then went on to explain this to the London hospital they in turn (and this will in the circumstances take a lot of believing).

If their criteria of brain removal was not met there may be a problem with conclusively summing up on Mark's death certificate that he had died of vCJD! The times have been, that when the brains were out the man would die, and there an end, with so many murders on their crowns, and push us from our stools, this is more strange, than such a murder is.

I was not impressed with the direction the hospital were trying to go since a previous MRI scan had shown clear pulvinar signs of prion damage way back in December 2005.

We agreed, that's my brother in law and myself that they could take a small slice of the white grey matter for research only and not to try and blackmail us this way, it was enough that they had researched Mark since January 2006 and written up about Mark's case in the medical journal The Lancet. And I wish Professor John Collinge the current lead in research in London's Prion Clinic of this horrific disease all the luck in the world in a cure albeit, that he once sat on the committee of SEAC and a lot of their decision making was highly controversial.

Our son's funeral was arranged for Thursday 25th May at the burial grounds of a cemetery in Brighton.

His autopsy scheduled for the previous day, the resulting death certificate issued a verdict of Variant creutzfeldt-Jacob disease.

And signed by the coroner for Brighton and Hove. Mr John Hooper, was duly registered in the Town Hall of Brighton.

Thursday 25th May 06: At nine in the morning of the day I was to bury my son I was running on autopilot, switching off any emotions that would get in the way of what I needed to accomplish, it was only now after our family had finally lost the battle that I could sense another dimension entering my every thought and I hated this intruder, I heard voices that were telling me go and seek justice for what has happened to your son, even at this early stage of bereavement.

My every thought and action was a guarded one, not wanting to be as open as I normally would be in any conversation.

I opened the car boot and loaded it up with chairs, I had driven to a synagogue hall in Hove and collected enough chairs for prayers after the funeral service, this was to take place in our mews house, and again a traditional conclusion to the burial ceremony.

My guarded emotions slipped as I stood outside the small synagogue hall that for generations had been used for final prayers by Jewish bereaved within the confines of our cemetery in Brighton and was about to receive Mark's coffin.

Through a mist of salty tears I watched as the black hearse carrying Mark's coffin came to a halt within feet of my numb body, how the hell can I bury my son it's all too soon, it should be me instead, an avalanche of anger and disbelief but within all of this a reluctant acceptance of the here and now, I have in truth been to many funerals but never seen one in 3D before.

So many people came to say their final farewells, I was unashamed of my tears not really caring how people portrayed me on this blacker than black day, the Rabbi spoke of Mark and what he knew of him and had learnt from others, from here it's again a tradition for chief mourners to remain seated in the synagogue hall before the grave ceremony and to be wished long life by friends and relations.

Finally my son's black draped coffin on its black trolley was eased to its black space with mourners closely following, to his final resting place of predominantly chalk and earth, and countless other gravestones marking only skeletal remains and long forgotten dreams, remember saying over and over to myself I am so sorry Mark, so sorry, I loved you so much. The coffin is lowered into a place where I will never be able to gaze on him again, a final prayer is said by me and I remember ably assisted by other good friends and then the grave back filled with Sussex chalk I initiated the proceedings, others then following including my eldest daughter's husband who in his valiant attempt to help fill the grave almost fell in himself but was rescued in time, my late son's body being hidden now from any further hurt in a place where we all have to go eventually, strangely Mark had died on May 23rd the exact same day as his late grandfather and was now buried just a short distance away in the same cemetery.

Leaving the cemetery we head back to the mews making sure the kettle is on, and sandwiches are cut, cakes displayed and the whiskey bottle and associated glasses are on display.

It is also traditional to cover any mirrors up in the house of mourning.

Early evening there is another service, in Jewish orthodox circles this service is marked by prayers normally at the family house of the deceased for seven nights it is called a Sheva (meaning 7 in Hebrew).

For any family a minimum of ten Jewish men need to be in attendance, we must have had a great deal more than that for not only was the house completely full but there was a large overspill in the mews itself, the service concluding with tea and cake, lots of wagging tongues, lots of people wishing us long life, they all being very supportive in their own way.

When everyone had gone my mind went back to the hearse and the black draped coffin and the very reason Mark was laid to rest so very much before his time, I remember kicking the garage door, but not remembering much else except hoping that time may heal the hurt that all of our family were feeling in May 2006.

For me it never did which is the main reason I needed to complete this book, despite some excellent counselling by Martlets Hospice after Mark's death which in truth I hung on to for over a year, all of our family were in desperate need of this and indeed as far as I am aware (although it isn't something that's my business) I believe my daughters are still attending occasional counselling sessions.

That's how much we hurt and we were all completely drained.

Monday 29th May 06: Although our son had been laid to rest in a Jewish Cemetery his own following for some time had been Buddhism, his years in Ipswich were enriched with this faith and a good deal of his leisure time spent learning as much as he could, attending various retreats and indeed his then girlfriend was of the same following.

It was felt important certainly by friends that the formal ceremony of Mark's burial on the previous Thursday should be followed by a Buddhist equivalent in Brighton.

And so it happened and all of this arranged magnificently by his friends.

Everybody who should have been there were there.

At 2.30 on Monday 29th May we all attended the Buddhist ceremony in Brighton.

Mark A Celebration.

Opened with acoustic guitar Blackbird - The Beatles. (Mark when he was well sang and accompanied himself on guitar to this lovely tune).

The Placing of flowers.

Introduction by Amarasiddhi.
Acoustic guitar – Somebody Loved - The Weepies.

Readings 2 Friends
Acoustic guitar. Wish you Were here – Pink Floyd

Readings other friends
Acoustic guitar Songbird-Eva Cassidy

Readings His two Sisters.
Song to be sung by all – DAYS – Kirsty MacColl

Lighting of Candles.

MARK
"Each friend represents a world in us. A world not possibly born until they arrive, and it is only by this meeting a new world is born."

Anais Nin

I don't believe there was a dry- eye in the house that afternoon.

We then all headed off to the Black Horse in Black Lion St in Brighton. I was still on autopilot.

There was an opportunity to write a little something down and my youngest daughter offered this to anyone who cared to. The following just a snapshot of that time when drinking to Mark now an absent friend.

Friend – tears and laughter, a combination Mark would have approved of xx.

Friend –it was beautiful. And, See you on MSN xx

It was a beautiful and enduring ceremony I've been honoured to be a part of Mark's life.

Sarah Perfect x Lucy T What a wonderful day for the one we loved so x .Louise. Mark told me there is even some hope in hopeless miss you great day.

Today's ceremony was the most expressive, poignant, sincere letting go ceremony I have ever been to, I'm so glad we had it for Mark. He was a man of sincerity and style and it suited his character perfectly.

A very special day. I felt Mark's calmness as I sung my heart out. Oh how I'll miss those sing songs with Mark xxx.

So there we have it, we all I suppose got on the bus, but had to leave Mark behind on our journey through life except he didn't want or ask for that!

Chapter Twelve

Picking Up The Pieces

On the 16th August 06 my late son had his Coroner's Inquest in Brighton.

We as a family had no legal representative present which was I think unfortunate, however I was able to cross examine one of the witnesses that took part in the inquest, he told the coroner that in 2004 when he advised Mark on his at risk status that he knew very little about vCJD, which poses two questions: Why then did the DOH refer Mark to this man in the first place; and secondly since he knew of his lack of knowledge in regard to the subject of variant CJD at that time, why did he not refer Mark on to a neurologist who did?

The same neurologist in 2006 said that our son had disappeared (quote) 'off his radar screen'. Not true, Mark remained at the same address, had the same job, same NHS no. Same Tel no.

Nothing contact ability wise had altered.

What did alter was his neurologist had moved on to a position with the Prion Clinic, under John Collinge in the Neurological Hospital in London's Queen Square. It was he who disappeared, Mark had effectively become isolated I prefer to call it abandoned to his GP who had an equally limited knowledge of CJD.

At the conclusion of our son's Coroner's Inquest the coroner was so moved as to write to the Department of Health, and as a direct result of that an 18 page report was published by the vCJD Clinical Governance Advisory Group, chaired by Sir William Stewart (An independent review for the Department of Health).

Just some of its recommendations are as follows: 'We recommend that the GP remains the clinical guardian and anchor of the healthcare needs of people at risk'.

'We recommend that the GP should be fully briefed, in ALL cases by a designated neurologist'.

'We recommend that the designated neurologist should then take the local clinical vCJD lead in assessing and providing advice, making contact with specialist services etc'.

'The condition of that person at risk should be reviewed if symptoms of concern develop'.

It is very plain to see that none of these events ever took place for our late son when they needed to be.

Thursday 17th August 2006 at 09.01: The Guardian newspaper reports; 'The government revealed yesterday it was reviewing the way it warns people they may be incubating the human form of Mad Cow Disease after transfusion with contaminated blood, as a coroner called for an urgent shake up in the present system.'

Pathetic, irresponsible, mal-aligned, and askew, were the Witches Within Westminster!!

Time after Time starting in 2003 in Mark's medical history.

20th May 2003- difficulty in concentrating

06 June 2003- lethargic

04June 2003- Tiredness, cognitive difficulties, poor concentration, poor functioning, having great difficulty with memory and recall.

September 2003- Anxious, Hypersomnia, no concentration, no memory, loses any thread of conversation.

By this time alarm bells should have been ringing, since only 12 weeks later he was told by the Department of Health that he may be at risk of vCJD!!!!!!!

This obvious link failed to get picked up.

A string of governmental errors (I can see now just why the present Tory Government want to sell off parts of the NHS to private concerns, they are obviously too incompetent to run it themselves.)

We wanted to try and make a difference, to raise awareness of vCJD, to educate the government and public about the massive shortcomings of the NHS Blood Transfusion Service including the enormous scandal of the many haemophiliacs who have been recipients of tainted blood products.

BBC cameras as well as ITV had captured us on camera telling the very sad story of what Mark and others had gone through. We had been reported in newspaper articles and on television news about the flaws and many mistakes of the government and its health ministers, of bungled decision making, and with that in mind I then decided in September 2006 to try a different tack.

I would ride my bike from Paris to London with a group of others to raise awareness about vCJD and a contaminated blood service in the UK, the ride from Paris along the Avenue Verte culminating in a VIP welcome on the Embankment in London would be reported in the media press.

I caught a ferry from Newhaven to Dieppe with others, then trained down to Paris, found our lodgings then after dining Al-Fresco an early night for the next day's journey.

Our starting point was the Notre Dame and we were accompanied by a very efficient guide and an assortment of French cyclists.

We made it back within three days and along the way a lot of the public were made more aware of the many shortfalls within the UK Blood Service, but it wasn't enough I needed to choose another path, a greater more meaningful one, that would give me and like minded supporters an opportunity to rectify and to modify the many failings that are still a part of our Blood Transfusion Service.

By now I was attending Martlets Hospice on a regular basis for counselling, although I am sure this did help psychologically, these visits back to Martlets were a strong reminder of Mark's passing in May of this year.

I was having vivid dreams of Mark nightly and it was so real, although in these dreams I knew he was gone it was sort of comforting to imagine briefly that my son was still alive; naughty but nice.

Strange I never thought that changing a light bulb would be a challenge.

Just had another 'tiff' with Eve, just one in a whole series of marital disputes about nothing in particular, the stress of losing our son really testing our marriage.

Eve didn't make her counselling session today so the counsellor rang me, I then in turn rang Eve, who said she couldn't face a session today, she sounded tearful and then switched her mobile off.

Ok she's hurting, I'm hurting, the whole bloody family is hurting but what can you do. And I kept saying to myself try and make something happen within the NHS Blood Service to improve the safety of this obviously very unsafe and floored component which should be above reproach!

My only escape was extracting my red racer from the garage, and clipping in, and feeling the sensual feeling of my body at one with my thoughts, a desire to drain my very soul it was almost a masochistic approach to searching for comfort anything that would take away a galaxy of haunting emotions of a pain that refused to leave me.

It's now February 2007 and we had arranged for a tree to be planted in one of Hove's synagogue grounds, a plaque was prepared in Mark's memory and on February 2nd a small ceremony was carried out by Rabbi Efune, the tree planted, the plaque mounted; a small token of our undying love for him.

May 27th 2007: In the Jewish religion it is customary to set the gravestone approximately one year after the burial, and so on this day we had invited friends and family back to Mark's final resting place.

Our family had been careful in choosing our son's marble stone, and both family and friends had chosen some beautiful words that had described their love for someone who had once been a star and I feel will be remembered for all of their lifetimes.

Prayers were said, a simple ceremony followed and memories stirred, a final goodbye I suppose to someone who had been a very special person.

June 2007 found me and a good friend boarding a plane for Inverness in Scotland complete with Road Bikes, Panniers, Rucksacks, we had planned to try and raise more awareness regarding NHS bloods with a ride from John o Grote's to Land's End.

The journey was testing but at the same time enjoyable, everyone we met on route sympathetic to the reasons we had for the ride. It took us two weeks covering over a thousand miles, our route coming down the west coast of Scotland through Bristol, Severn Bridge, Somerset, Devon, Cornwall proudly wearing a T-shirt displaying the reasons for the trip we finally arrived at our destination in a Rainstorm in Land's End and welcomed the bath and evening meal. The ride proved to be a very therapeutic one for me if only because it was physically challenging and channelled the main body of my thoughts into survival mode and I was on a mission, to complete this journey my inner thoughts, were a voice from Mark, smiling and encouraging his dad on every revolution of the bike's eccentric chain rings.

Although a very worthwhile way of trying to raise awareness and it had been publicised well by our local news media I had this strong feeling as we trained our way back to Brighton that I needed another strategy to discover a fresher and more divisive approach in headlining the massive problem within our blood service, a problem that the government was not addressing with any particular conviction it appeared to me.

And in between the leg cramps that seemed to be gathering pace on board our chattanogachoochoo back to a Mosquito less Brighton (Scotland has its fair share of sporran clad mosquitoes) my considered view was this; TV interviews, Press reviews, letters to Downing Street and generally to get the subject highlighted just of course as it should be, the downside was would I be as sufficiently as hot a chestnut for little me to make a difference? Probably not. But if there were more like minded people, enough to increase pressure on the Government to embarrass them for their lack of purpose then maybe.

All that thought lost to our train pulling in to Brighton Station and unloading our two wheeled companions who like us needed a bed for the night and their tyres inflated a tad.

It seemed I slept very well since I awoke to have breakfast at lunch time.

April 2008 saw our family at Sussex University, having previously made an arrangement with the appropriate authorities within the university to have a suitable tree planted, to incorporate a suitably inscribed plaque, and in addition a plaqued bench in the grounds of Mark's ex-university. We found comfort in this dedication and in Spring and Summer I often found myself sitting on this bench and in my mind's eye see Mark carrying his lecture notes through the grounds towards the library. With my red road bike supported by Mark's dedicated seat of rest I allowed my imagination to run free, I was then waiting for him to finish his semester, my bike was replaced by a very smart VW Cabriolet and we would return to Hove, driving up Coldean Lane a steep hill that lay adjacent to his university, and surrounded with my childhood memories of youthful innocence and optimism, to return him safely to the bosom of his family. I reached across but only felt my water bottle in its carrier on my silent red painted ever patient bike, the car had been replaced like my late son with an ending that no one would want either in their Xmas stocking or indeed in their worst nightmare.

I remember the day we had that dedication, it was snowing hard, a picture postcard setting in the beautiful setting of Stanmer Park an area I grew up in as a young boy, little did I know years later how sad and reflective I would one day be in that setting knowing we had all lost an important part of who we were, a part of our lives that was irreplaceable.

There are three benches dedicated to my late son's memory, one of which sits in the grounds of the BT's main Research and Development Building at Martlesham Heath, Ipswich where our son worked until he became too ill.

The second on Brighton's seafront opposite the very attractive bandstand its inscription reads: 'Mark Buckland, he loved the sea and the sky'.

And the third in the grounds of Sussex University.

Yesterday has now gone for our family, to be replaced with tears and a melancholy that hums its tune soulfully in my head night and day, writing provides little solace except the forlorn hope that maybe someone reading this may briefly share my burden, my broken heart will remain I fear, all the time I have breath in me.

It's now December 2011 and despite two or more visits to no 10 Downing Street handing in letters pleading with our government to address the blood services inadequacies, meetings within Westminster, and the many other times I have met with current advisory committees on bloods, then times we as a body have marched on Westminster carrying plaques saying 'Make BLOOD SAFE' nothing seems to have moved forward.

The Witches Within Westminster seem untroubled.

For the ingredients of their Cauldron.

This has always been the rhetoric on which all co-defendants of the question when put to them regarding Mark's undetected symptoms from 2003 say: 'vCJD has an insidious clinical onset and it's early features, for example depression, anxiety, personality changes and sensory disturbances are highly non-specific. It is therefore difficult to diagnose early (in the absence of another reason to suspect this diagnosis). However monitoring of high risk groups such as recipients of blood transfusions from a donor who developed vCJD should allow it's recognition at an early stage'.

These stylized, impassive, defensive, answers, simply confirm their guilt at not being able to answer truthfully or indeed ever think they are fit for purpose.

But there was an early stage in April 2000 when the Department of Health knew Mark was at risk from one of his blood donors but decided to say nothing and furthermore when they eventually did they totally ignored their own warning! Mark was displaying all of these symptoms at a stage before and after their eventual warning letter which was sent in December 2003. There was a reason but it was ignored, and this is justice (Oh really)?

Clearly the decision makers within the Department of Health at that time were as the saying goes 'on another planet', but poor decisions cost lives and that needs addressing. I sincerely hope this true story may make a difference to the present shortcomings of our NHS Blood Transfusion Service but I somehow doubt that. On my last visit to Westminster I had an arranged meeting with representatives of SABTO (the safety advisory committee on blood, tissue and organs), on where the government were, on safety standards within the Blood Transfusion Service. I was accompanied by a mother who had also lost her son to vCJD, the human form of BSE. That was more than 3 years ago and to date nothing has changed to make it safer! After the meeting we walked arm in arm as we made our way towards the exit doors, down a myriad of grey steps matching exactly our grey thoughts where I imagined I heard the chilling whispers from the wayward sisters and their master Hecate, of whom Shakespeare wrote, and from the cavernous corridors of Westminster's Victorian cathedral like Emporium, the Brindled cat issued its muted meow, both of us now tearful, because we somehow knew nothing positive would come about, although I couldn't see any witches' cat, it seemed that in every corner of the building the shadows that were cast were trying to hide years of poor and maligned policy decision making, but failed to hide the pain that would now always be with us.

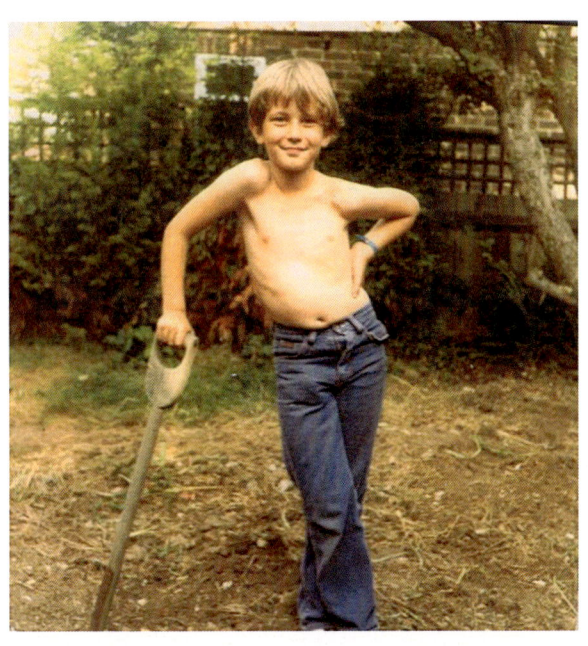
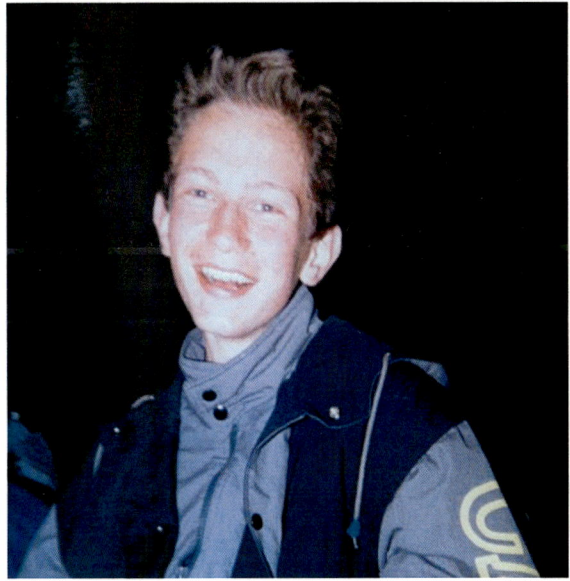

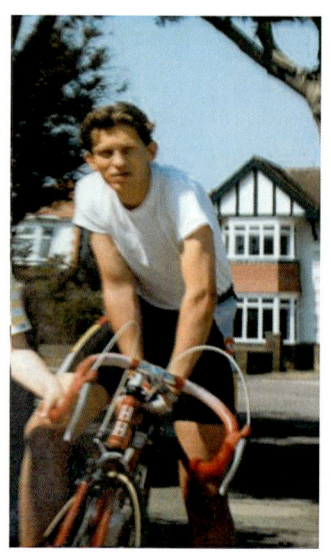
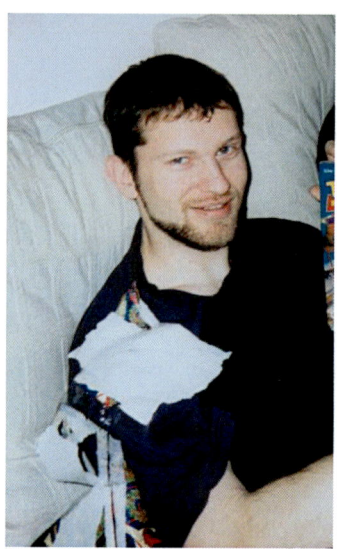
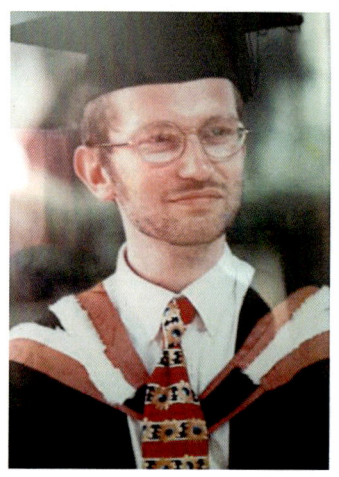
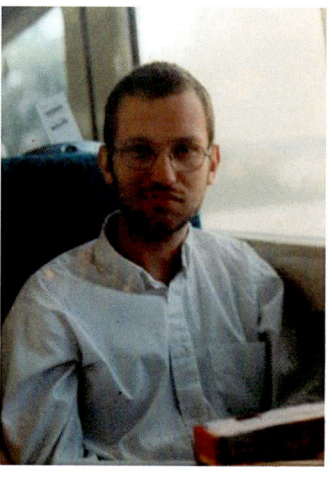

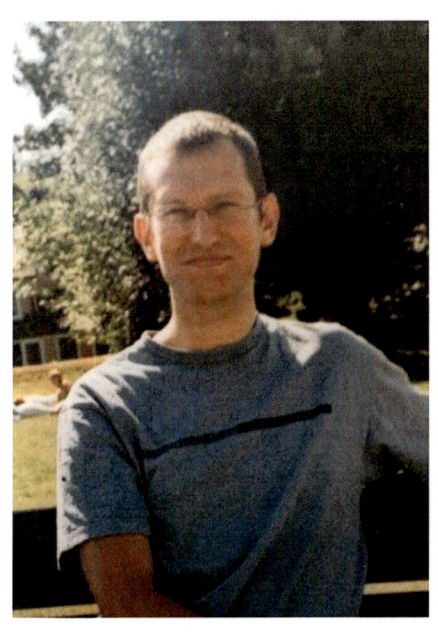

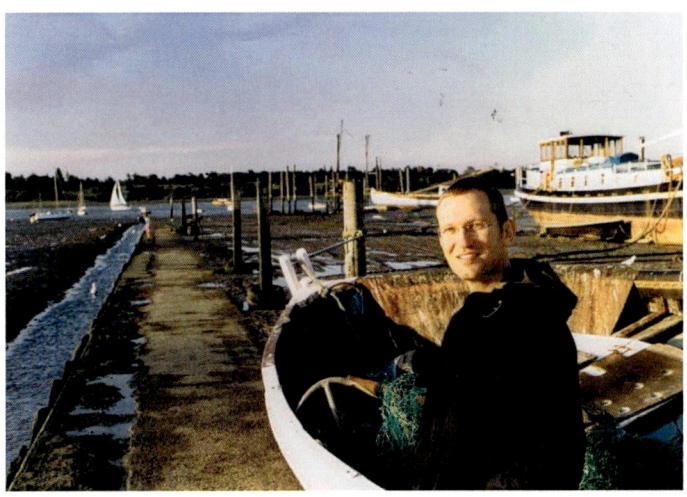

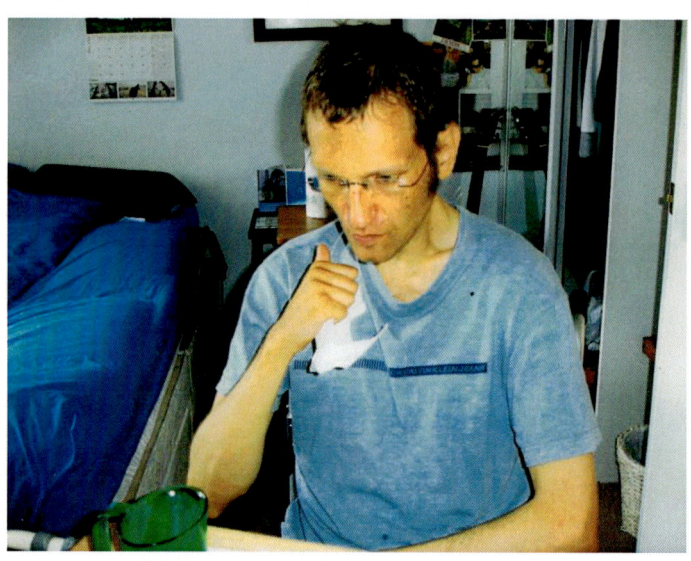

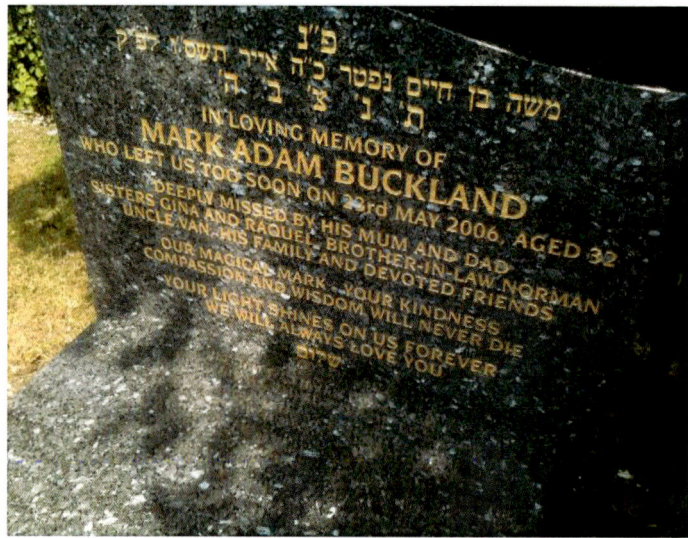

On Mark's gravestone the following words:

**I am not gone but merely walk within you
Listen to my footfall in your heart.**

Afterword

It would be disrespectful of me not to mention even at the conclusion of this book the work and research of the late Mark Purdey, who wrote an inspiring Book called 'Animal Pharm' on his findings on Governmental failings within The Ministry of Agriculture and Fisheries! His criticisms on the administration of toxic organophosphates and pesticides, it was to me a breath of fresh air to expose and reveal the total inadequate partner relationship between government and pharmaceutical companies between government and food manufacturers who looked only to swell profits by muscling in on agriculture, shame on you for not reading and inwardly digesting the late Rachael Carson's book 'Silent Spring!'

And finally all of these health scares continue, we are now in 2013 and are finding horse meat that is sold as 100% beef, a blood supply that still falls desperately short of being safe, people still dying of vCJD, and it will continue because more attention is paid to big fat profits within the food industry and government than to safeguards within them. We all need to realise that Organic Farming is the way forward after all it's simply common sense!

THE END